Clinical Research in Practice: A Guide for the Bedside Scientist

Janet Houser, PhD, RN
Department of Health Services Administration
Regis University
Denver, CO

Joanna Bokovoy, DrPH, RN
Director, Healthcare Research
Lehigh Valley Hospital and Health Network
Allentown, PA

JONES AND BARTLETT PUBLISHERS
Sudbury, Massachusetts
BOSTON   TORONTO   LONDON   SINGAPORE

World Headquarters

Jones and Bartlett Publishers	Jones and Bartlett Publishers	Jones and Bartlett Publishers
40 Tall Pine Drive	Canada	International
Sudbury, MA 01776	6339 Ormindale Way	Barb House, Barb Mews
978-443-5000	Mississauga, Ontario L5V 1J2	London W6 7PA
info@jbpub.com	Canada	UK
www.jbpub.com		

Jones and Bartlett's books and products are available through most bookstores and online booksellers. To contact Jones and Bartlett Publishers directly, call 800-832-0034, fax 978-443-8000, or visit our website, www.jbpub.com.

Substantial discounts on bulk quantities of Jones and Bartlett's publications are available to corporations, professional associations, and other qualified organizations. For details and specific discount information, contact the special sales department at Jones and Bartlett via the above contact information or send an email to specialsales@jbpub.com.

ISBN-13: 978-0-7637-3875-4
ISBN-10: 0-7637-3875-1

Library of Congress Cataloging-in-Publication Data

Houser, Janet, 1954-
  Clinical research in practice : a guide for the bedside scientist / Janet
Houser, Joanna Bokovoy.
     p. ; cm.
  Includes bibliographical references and index.
  ISBN-13: 978-0-7637-3875-4 (pbk. : alk. paper)
  ISBN-10: 0-7637-3875-1 (pbk. : alk. paper)
  1. Clinical medicine—Research.   I. Bokovoy, Joanna. II. Title.
  [DNLM: 1. Health Services Research—methods. 2. Clinical Nursing
Research—methods. 3. Research Design.   W 84.3 H842c 2006]
  R850.H677 2006
  616.0072—dc22
                                    2006001439

6048

The authors, editor, and publisher have made every effort to provide accurate information. However, they are not responsible for errors, omissions, or for any outcomes related to the use of the contents of this book and take no responsibility for the use of the products described. Treatments and side effects described in this book may not be applicable to all patients; likewise, some patients may require a dose or experience a side effect that is not described herein. The reader should confer with his or her own physician regarding specific treatments and side effects. Drugs and medical devices are discussed that may have limited availability controlled by the Food and Drug Administration (FDA) for use only in a research study or clinical trial. The drug information presented has been derived from reference sources, recently published data, and pharmaceutical research data. Research, clinical practice, and government regulations often change the accepted standard in this field. When consideration is being given to use of any drug in the clinical setting, the healthcare provider or reader is responsible for determining FDA status of the drug, reading the package insert, reviewing prescribing information for the most up-to-date recommendations on dose, precautions, and contraindications, and determining the appropriate usage for the product. This is especially important in the case of drugs that are new or seldom used.

Production Credits

Acquisitions Editor: Kevin Sullivan	Manufacturing Buyer: Amy Bacus
Production Director: Amy Rose	Composition: Graphic World
Associate Editor: Amy Sibley	Cover Design: Timothy Dziewit
Production Editor: Carolyn F. Rogers	Printing and Binding: Malloy, Inc.
Marketing Manager: Emily Ekle	Cover Printing: Malloy, Inc.

Printed in the United States of America
13 12   10 9 8 7 6 5 4

DEDICATION

In memory of my mom, Marty Houser—
My first and best teacher, inspiration, and friend

In honor of my dad, Alex Bokovoy, MD, FACS—
As a father, surgeon, and scientist, you continually inspire,
support, and challenge me

Table of Contents

Appendices

Foreword

When one thinks of a scientist, the picture of a white lab coat–clad individual standing amid microscopes, chemicals, and Petri dishes in a laboratory setting might emerge. One might picture the individual working alone amid scientific formulas and experiments, discovering cures for the many diseases that we see in our daily practice.

As healthcare students, clinicians, and professionals, we know that research to determine best practice is a necessity in our environment. We know that our practice environments are our laboratories, with questions waiting to be asked and practices begging to be challenged. Gone are the days when we perform an intervention simply because that was the way it was always done. In its place is the reality that the continued advancement of our healthcare practice is dependent on our knowledge of the evidence—the scientific basis of our care.

Patients, families, and communities deserve the practice changes and interventions that have emerged from research done in our laboratories, our practice environments. To add to our body of knowledge, to advance our healthcare practices, and to apply our knowledge for the advancement of patient and family care requires not only an appreciation for research, but also an involvement in research by those providing the care, those that have the questions and understand the impact that answers can bring.

We all must be students of research. Developing a habit of inquiry, not settling for the status quo, and seeking even more effective means to treat patients are important to any profession. An environment of inquiry, the encouragement of questions, and the constant search for best practices are hallmarks of magnet hospitals. Preparing to practice in environments of this nature requires the development of respect for research and an appreciation for evidence-based practice.

Actually learning the concepts of research may seem onerous. The authors have taken research and evidence-based concepts and presented them in such a manner as to create enthusiasm and spark interest to advance patient care and enhance your commitment to research as a professional. They have shown that conducting applied clinical research is attainable and can be accomplished by providers of care, with guidance from those skilled in research.

The authors begin by discussing the role of research in clinical practice and then lead you through a step-by-step guide to research in practice. From the determination of a question through the application of results, you will be led through the process in a manner that is logical and easily understandable. Along the way, you will be stimulated to think. The fear of research will be eased, and the potential for your involvement will be enhanced.

Performing research and applying the results to help patients and families achieve effective health outcomes are the reasons that we become professionals. No satisfaction is as great as making a difference in the life of another. Appreciation for, conducting, and then applying research results will allow you to make that difference.

Terry Capuano, RN, MSN, MBA
Senior Vice President, Clinical Services
Lehigh Valley Hospital and Health Network (Magnet designated since August 2002)

Preface

The aim of this book is to help the bedside scientist find, understand, and use clinical research. We have used the term *bedside scientist* because it is our belief that some of the most useful patient care research is conducted in the living laboratories that are our clinical settings. The book's usefulness is not limited to those at the bedside, however; every healthcare practitioner needs to understand and contribute to the body of knowledge that is the basis for clinical practice. For a long time in health care, scientific research was left to academics. This no longer works in health care. The contemporary healthcare environment makes every clinician accountable for determining the value of his or her interventions.

Although much has been gained from basic and theoretical healthcare research, practice-based research has lagged far behind. As a result, many bedside clinicians' research skills have become rusty, and the thought of designing a research project—even a small, focused study—can seem daunting. This book is intended to help the bedside scientist take a study from question, to design, to practice in as painless a way as possible.

In our workshops for clinical practitioners, we have discovered no shortage of research books available for clinicians and have also heard from our students and clients that many scholarly books are too complicated, in-depth, and technical for the clinician who has little time to sift through hundreds of pages of text. We have designed this book to be a straightforward, reader-friendly approach to a complex subject, thus hopefully arming the clinician with the information that he or she needs to become engaged in the research process.

The book begins with an overview of the importance of research for bedside scientists and then introduces a step-by-step approach to reading research and designing focused research studies. Each step is explained in detail in the chapters that follow. We have included a chapter that is an overview of survey and qualitative designs—often ignored in the evidence-based practice effort, but valuable nonetheless in dealing with the human condition. Our final chapter gives suggestions for communicating the results of bedside science studies in a way that contributes to the greater professional body of knowledge. The appendix includes some helpful reference tools, including a glossary of common research terms, an example of an informed consent, and a survey instrument. To illustrate the appraisal process, we present a research article and walk through the evaluative steps with this real-world example.

The chapters have side boxes that are intended to help the reader understand and use good research processes. Each chapter begins with a brief overview that helps the reader to determine quickly whether the content will apply to their research efforts. The chapters might also include the following:

- *From the mouths of bedside scientists:* Clinicians are often in the best position to explain research concepts to other clinicians, and we have asked students, colleagues, and bedside scientists to do so here.
- *Where to look:* Half of the problem in evaluating all of the parts of a research article is finding them in a lengthy and complicated article. We simplify the process by directing the reader to the most likely locations for each research element in a typical article.
- *Hitting the stacks:* Translating research concepts to their representation in the literature can be frustrating; we use excerpts from published articles to illustrate how key concepts might look.
- *Strengthen your practice:* We suggest ways a busy clinician can apply the principles in this book to practice-based research in a realistic way that does not compromise the quality of the result.
- *Another way to look at it:* We have found in our workshops that stories can simplify the complicated aspects of research and create understanding through analogies. Most of these illustrations are not from health care, but rather from life, and use examples that anyone can appreciate.
- *For more depth and detail:* We have used our experiences as a basis for the text in this book, and thus, no citations exist in the body of the text. The general references that we used, as well as additional references that might be of help to the reader, are included here instead.
- *Concepts in action:* These sections use real-life research to illustrate and illuminate the important concepts of practice-based research. Each is a description of a real-life bedside science research project—warts and all. Some of these describe an entire study from beginning to end, pointing out ways that original plans had to be modified to fit reality. Some describe multiple ways to approach the same problem and show that there are, indeed, many ways to accomplish quality bedside science projects.

- *Evaluation checklists:* Evaluation checklists are included to help the reader focus his or her appraisal on the most important characteristics when reading research. In Appendix 4, all of these checklists have been aggregated into a single list to provide the reader with a summary tool for evaluating the quality of an article.

It is our hope that this book will serve as a guide, providing uncomplicated direction for the complicated process of using research in practice. It is also our hope that the book will inspire bedside scientists—whether they are still students or practicing—to create scientific evidence for their own practices.

Acknowledgments

The authors thank the contributors who wrote substantive parts of this text. Julie Jones, RN, MSN, wrote the Concepts in Action for Chapter 9, and Sheila Carlon, PhD, RHIA, FAHIMA, wrote the section of Chapter 5 that deals with the complex issues raised by HIPAA. We both gratefully acknowledge Terry Capuano, RN, MSN, for writing the Foreword and for all of her support in this endeavor. A special thanks goes to Patricia Ladewig, PhD, for her thoughtful mentorship throughout this project, and to Floyd Ott for creating all of the figures for the book.

Deepest thanks go to Kathy Baker, RN, MPH and Mark Young, MD (in memoriam) who partnered with Dr. Bokovoy in founding the Lehigh Valley Hospital Bedside Scientist Institute for improved patient outcomes, and whose graduates provided many of the research examples used in this book. Lehigh Valley Hospital Clinical Services leadership and staff provided invaluable support of this project in ways too numerous to list. Special appreciation goes to those bedside scientists who were members of the multidisciplinary teams that designed and who carried out the research reported in the Concepts in Action, including the following:

- Chapter 2: Unpublished study by Bedside Scientists. Kosman, B., N. Dirico, and J. Bokovoy.
- Chapter 3: Biswas, A.K., D.A. Bruce, F.H. Sklar, J.L. Bokovoy, and J.F. Sommerauer. (2002). Treatment of acute traumatic brain injury in children with moderate hypothermia improves intracranial hypertension. *Critical Care Medicine* 30(12): 2742–51.
- Chapter 4: Seislove, E., and M. Pasquale. Mild traumatic brain injury protocol. (Unpublished).
- Chapter 6: Brenner, S., J. Boucher, L. Gogel, H. Hettel, V. Rupp, S. Dreher, J. Christman, P. Matula, and J. Bokovoy. Randomized, placebo-

controlled study using LMX4 to decrease pain during urgent venipuncture in children. (Unpublished).

- Chapter 7: Unpublished studies by Bedside Scientists. Gogle, J., J. Waller, D. Belles, E. Linden, L. Rusch, V. Brancato, O. Rust, and J. Bokovoy. (Labor and delivery workflow study). Matchett, S., K. Baker, and J. Bokovoy. (ICU nurse workflow study). Brenner, S., K. Burdett, A. Brown, and J. Bokovoy. (The effects of parent–physician relationships on the recovery of hospitalized children with bronchiolitis). Sacco, E., Z. Mawji, K. Casey, and J. Bokovoy. (Impact of a new hydrophilic straight catheter on UTI). Sabella, V., K. Miller, L. Cornman, J. Novak, K. Gonzalez, L. Baga., S. O'Neill, T. Englehardt, and J. Bokovoy. (Comparison of two ventilators on patient outcomes).
- Chapter 8: Unpublished studies by Bedside Scientists. Barber, J., L. Geraci, L. Karper, and J. Bokovoy. (Use of music on anxiety in psychiatric patients). Palmer, E., J. Benninger, M. Leshko, V. Trexler, and L. Engel. (Physician–patient communication). Strawdinger, J., L. Snyder, D. Gotthardt, and C. Dempsey. (Rest in the ICU). Published study. Lequier, L., H. Nikaidoh, S. Leonard, J. Bokovoy, M. White, P. Scannon, and B. Giroir. (2000). Preoperative and postoperative endotoxemia in children with congenital heart disease. *Chest* 117: 1706–12.
- Chapter 10: Published study. Panik, A., J. Bokovoy, B. Karoly, K. Badillo, C. Buckenmyer, C. Vose, J. Wheary, G. Sierzega, L. Deitrick, and A. Hyduke. (2006). Research on the frontlines of healthcare—A cooperative learning approach. *Nursing Research*. (This study also appeared in Chapter 7).
- Appendix 1—A Sample Informed Consent Form: Brenner, S., K. Burdett, A. Brown, and J. Bokovoy. The effects of parent–physician relationships on the recovery of hospitalized children with bronchiolitis. (Unpublished).
- Appendix 2—A Survey Example: Trapasso, J., E. Sacco, D. Arnold, and J. Bokovoy. Patient evaluation of hospitalization for radical prostatectomy. (Unpublished).

Part I

An Introduction to Bedside Science

CHAPTER 1

The Role of Research in Clinical Practice

In this chapter, you will learn to

- Distinguish the value of research in contemporary clinical practice
- Make the connection between research and professionalism
- Get involved in practice-based research activities
- Recognize the similarity between quality projects and practice-based research
- Identify the benefits of participating on a clinical research team

In professional journals, the words research and science and evidence seem to appear everywhere. While listening to another news program that describes the devastating but unknown side effects of a drug or how a commonly accepted approach to care does not really work, you consider why research is so valuable in making life better. Research used to be something that was done in a laboratory; a researcher or scientist never touched a patient. Now research is an integral part of clinical practice. Research is everywhere: in the news, on the internet, as the highlight of every clinical or management conference, and quoted by your patients. It is no longer sacred, which is probably good. You know enough about research, however, to understand that a certain level of knowledge and skill must precede any research undertaking.

When you think about it, seeking evidence as a basis for practice is not anything new. Clinical care began with researchers and scientists such as Hippocrates, who is considered the father of

3

medicine and who wrote, "Declare the past, diagnose the present, foretell the future; practice these acts. As to diseases, make a habit of two things—to help, or at least to do no harm." Of course, science is how we know what will help and hopefully will do no harm. Other pioneer medical researchers come to mind—James Lind, who found that eating citrus fruit prevented scurvy; Robert Boyle, whose investigation of gas and pressure led to modern-day pulmonary science; Florence Nightingale, whose work with medical statistics was so impressive that she was elected to membership in the Statistical Society of England.

*Professional journal articles are full of empirical references, and terms such as **p value**, **t-test**, **r-squared**, **coefficient alpha**, and **power analysis** are common. You are proud of the fact that you know the rudiments of research analysis and are beginning to understand what most of them mean.*

It is becoming clear that quality clinical care and research go hand in hand. You now realize that a better understanding of research makes you a better clinician. You also know that similar to clinical practice, research takes time and practice to learn well. You have read enough that you are thinking of research questions that you would like to study; now you are even toying with the idea of doing your own research. You would like to know that your own practice is based on the best possible evidence and that you are making a contribution to the body of knowledge that is the basis of your profession. Where should you start? You know that it is important—you want to be involved. Somehow, you know that this is half of the battle.

The focus on evidence as a basis for clinical practice is truly a focus on research. Research is a systematic approach to answering questions, a disciplined method for solving problems based on objective evidence. Research is at the root of professionalism; it confirms that all clinical disciplines have a close connection to a scientific foundation. Using scientific evidence as a basis for practice seems straightforward—in fact, it is assumed that clinical practices have their roots in empirically derived knowledge. This is not a simple issue, however, because research skills have taken a back seat to clinical skills in health care for some time. Some of this phenomenon is due to the shortage of skilled clinical practitioners; when there is more work than can be done with existing staff, clinical tasks come first. Some is due to a reduced emphasis on research in educational curricula that already have too much material to cover. Some is due to cost controls in health care that limit access to research databases, statistical experts, and the time needed to design and conduct research.

In spite of these challenges, quality clinical care requires a clinician to develop skills as a bedside scientist, with the ability to read, evaluate, use, and conduct focused research studies. It is equally clear that research knowledge may be a rusty and unused skill set for many clinicians. The thought of relearning the steps of the scientific method can be daunting for bedside scientists who are more interested in immediate application of findings than in theoretical musings.

One of the challenges of applied clinical research is that sometimes there is the concern that to be a good researcher you must also be a skilled research scientist and statistician. This keeps many bedside scientists from pursuing a research agenda and is the wrong reason for avoiding research. Expecting that all bedside scientists have research design and statistical expertise can be likened to an expectation that all clinicians have proficiency in multiple specialties. We would all quickly agree that this would be an unreasonable expectation. When a clinician is expected to function in an unfamiliar specialty, he or she is provided with consultants and support people to help him or her succeed. The same can be said for clinical research. Consulting with research designers and statisticians is an expected part of the research process. One of the best models for doing good practice-based research is a partnership between a clinician and a research or statistical expert.

This does not negate the need for clinicians to have a basic understanding of research and statistics. Clinicians still need a fundamental understanding of statistics to read and evaluate research studies and to work effectively with their collaborators. This book helps clinicians learn the most important research concepts to understand and apply the research they read, and to conduct a bedside science research project.

THE VALUE OF RESEARCH

The value of research is profound. It helps us to weed out truth from error and separate evidence from anecdote and science from myth. It relies on empiricism rather than eloquence to make a rational argument. Patients trust that we provide the best possible care based on the best available evidence. Research studies give you that evidence; it is essential for continued improvement in patient care processes. If the clinician relies on chance or anecdote alone to determine that a treatment or procedure is effective, unwitting harm can occur. At the very least, a patient's time and efforts may be wasted. Evidence-based practice is patient-centered care at its best and simply means that the clinician first finds and evaluates the best available evidence and then

From the Mouths of Bedside Scientists: How Clinicians Talk About Practice-Based Research

Why should we base our practice on research evidence?
We should base our practice on research as much as possible because then we can trust that what we are doing is really quality care. . . . I would definitely feel more confident with my clinical care if I knew that research backed it up.

Time is such a huge issue when you take care of patients, and the more we study what we do, the easier it will be to prioritize the way we focus our time in the care of our patients. It is possible that much of what we do does not need to be done.

Why is research evidence important in clinical practice?
Research gives validation to what we do as health professionals. In order to show the effectiveness of what we do, it is imperative to demonstrate that what we do works and accomplishes our goals. Research gives us direction for future practice and support for current practice.

In my experience, the best practices come from research founded on a true desire to improve the quality of patient care. Accepting what has always been done as a standard of practice is not always the best for our patients. Looking for new studies that will result in positive outcomes for our patients is always a good idea.

Research is essentially a type of problem solving with a specific set of rules. Whenever a scientist is confounded with a problem that has no available solution, he or she looks to the research to find an answer. Research provides us with solutions to problems for which no answer existed in the past.

takes into consideration the patient's personal preferences and the clinician's expertise in deciding on a final plan of care.

Unfortunately, except in drug and device studies, the best evidence often takes years to make it to clinical practice. Much of what we do for our patients has no evidence to back it up. Thus, it is up to the clinician to not only provide what they "think" is the best care, but also find or create evidence that demonstrates that they *are* providing the best possible care. Specific clinical actions need to be solidly based on scientific evidence so that we can assure that those actions are clinically appropriate and cost-effective, and lead to desirable outcomes. Research knowledge and skills elevate and advance each clinical profession.

PROFESSIONALISM AND RESEARCH

Research goes hand in hand with professionalism. Professionalism is at its most fundamental an accountability to patients—taking action that is in their best interest. Reflect on your patients. They "know" research. They have read the latest research on the Internet and in magazines and newspapers. They have heard how Uncle John's involvement in a research study saved his life. Research has meaning to them. Thus, when they ask you why you are not treating them with treatment A, your evidence-based response will possibly impress them more than "I think that this treatment would work better for you because of my experiences with my other patients like you."

Many of your clinical colleagues are already familiar with research terms, and many have done research. Your research knowledge and expertise gives you the chance to speak with them as a peer and learn things that could change the way that you care for your patients. It can also be the opportunity for you to teach a colleague who has less understanding and knowledge of research. Clinicians with research expertise and knowledge can best lead the way for the highest quality of care for patients.

Think about how evidence has led to changes in cardiac care. Methods for administering cardiopulmonary resuscitation have changed dramatically over the last 2 decades as a result of research on outcomes. Manual intervention has been supplanted by research that indicates that defibrillation is more effective. Now a portable defibrillator can be used to evaluate the heart rhythm, or lack thereof, and provide the necessary treatment at the scene. The more quickly this defibrillation is administered the better—research shows that for every minute after sudden cardiac arrest happens, the odds of the person surviving decreases by 7% to 10%. Using current evidence, it appears that early defibrillation could increase survival rates to 30% or more. Circulation to the vital organs returns more quickly, and the patient will probably have better outcomes. This good thing will improve lives.

BEDSIDE SCIENTIST ROLES IN RESEARCH

The bedside scientist may be an effective team member on any number of research projects. The roles of a bedside scientist relative to research are not limited to participating in actual studies, however. The professional clinician has responsibilities to use research in a variety of ways to improve practice.

Most bedside scientists are first exposed to clinical research as *informed consumers*. The informed consumer of research is able to find appropriate research studies, to read them critically, to evaluate their findings for validity,

Strengthen Your Research Role

Very few bedside scientists start their research career by designing independent research. Most researchers start by becoming familiar with the research of others and seeking out opportunities to learn more about the process. You can strengthen your research role in a variety of ways:

- Read research routinely. If you do not subscribe to professional journals, make it a habit to visit the medical library regularly and leaf through articles. Become familiar with the way research is conducted and reported. Commit to read and critique at least one research study a month.
- Join a professional journal club. Journal clubs give you the opportunity to read and critique research in a group setting and to learn from the other members of the club. If your health care organization does not have a journal club, start one.
- Volunteer to participate in the development of a clinical practice guideline through a systematic review process. You will learn how to define a research question, conduct a methodical literature search, and evaluate studies for validity. Systematic reviews involve reading a large number of studies; thus, you will get a lot of experience in a short period of time and will be able to make a contribution to clinical practice in the process.
- Get involved in quality studies that are quantitative in nature. Many of the skills needed for quantitative quality studies are similar to those used for practice-based research and give you the opportunity to learn statistical analytic methods.
- Seek out educational opportunities and research conferences to improve your research skills. Talk to researchers who have similar interests to yours, and look for studies that you can replicate on a smaller scale.
- Actively participate in data collection, as either a collector or a subject. Involvement in either will give you ideas about how reliability is maintained and threats to validity are controlled.

and to use the findings in practice. Bedside scientists may also participate in *research-related activity*. These activities may include journal clubs or groups that meet periodically to critique research studies. Attending research presentations and discussing posters at conferences also expose the bedside scientist to a variety of research studies.

As the bedside scientist gets more proficient in the research process, involvement in a *systematic review* is a logical next step. A systematic review results in an evidence-based practice guideline and requires the ability to develop research questions, to write inclusion criteria, to conduct in-depth literature searches, and to critique the results of many studies. This participation also leads to facilitating changes in clinical practice on a larger scale and requires the bedside scientist to use leadership and communication skills.

Involvement in actual research studies does not require complete control or in-depth design abilities. *Assisting with data collection* can take the form of helping measure outcomes on subjects or personally performing as a good subject. Clinicians are frequently recruited to participate in studies; in this way you assure that your practice is represented. Collecting data for the studies of other researchers can give you valuable insight into methods that are used to assure reliability and control threats to validity, which help in designing your own experiments.

Most bedside scientists do not immediately start with an individual research study but *serve on a research team*. As part of a team, you can learn the skills needed to conduct research while relying on the expertise of a group of individuals. Serving on a team gives you the opportunity to participate in research in a collegial way, collaborating with others to achieve a mutual goal.

The most advanced bedside scientists are *producers of research*, designing and conducting their own research projects. An individual is rarely able to accomplish a research project on his or her own; thus, you will more likely lead a research team. This requires research and analytic skills and also skills in leading groups, managing projects, and soliciting organizational commitment.

QUALITY OF CARE AND RESEARCH

Research infuses quality into practice. Most health care organizations have some type of quality department because better quality means better outcomes. Projects defined as "Quality Improvement" and "Process Improvement" are frequently carried out in health care organizations but are rarely considered research projects. This is an erroneous approach. Quality-improvement studies use a systematic method to evaluate data about processes and outcomes and recommend interventions—much like practice-based research projects. Research methods should be applied to either of these to give the best possible understanding of the problem and how to make it better.

Quality-improvement and practice-based research have much in common. Both are systematic, rigorous processes based on disciplined inquiry. Quality-improvement studies start with the investigation of a process with a goal of reducing variation; research starts with investigation of a phenomenon with a goal of improving outcomes. Quality improvement is used to explain how processes are performing in quantitative ways; research is used to differentiate the effects of interventions in quantitative ways. Quality improvement results in a change in practice to improve outcomes—in this way, it is identical to practice-based research.

One major difference between quality studies and practice-based research relates to the Health Information Portability and Accountability Act (HIPAA). These requirements for data protection apply to identifiable, patient-level data, but most quality studies get a special institutional review board (IRB) waiver that allows the investigators to study patient data without having to get consent on each patient. No such waiver exists for practice-based research, and thus, the IRB is a major consideration during design. IRB and HIPAA requirements are discussed in detail in Chapter 5.

COLLABORATING WITH COLLEAGUES

In the clinical arena, research is often a team sport for a variety of reasons. A multidisciplinary team best answers many questions. Most quality concerns benefit from a multidisciplinary perspective. Working with a team can help to lessen the workload of a research project and address the challenge of finding adequate time to design and carry out the study. For example, when you first begin thinking about research ideas, sharing the idea with colleagues from a variety of clinical disciplines can give you quick—and sometimes creative—perspectives. As you focus the idea into a question, colleagues can help you refine the question because they will each be looking at it from a different viewpoint. Another outcome of a strong research team is a system of checks and balances to assure that nothing is missed and that every aspect of the study is carefully done.

The support provided by a team approach goes beyond the legwork needed to carry out the study. It could be termed *moral support*. It is that feeling that you are not facing the challenge of research alone. It puts a collegial, collaborative face on the research process. Knowing that others understand and share what it takes to do research is a help.

For example, a researcher interested in studying factors that increase the length of stay in a critical care unit will be more successful if he or she involves medical staff, nursing personnel, nutritionists, respiratory therapists, pharmacists, and other therapists. Each professional brings to the team unique knowledge and perspective on the problem being studied. Having a variety of professionals spreads the workload associated with the study and gives rise to more opportunities to communicate about the research project. Without a team, practice-based research is almost impossible for one person to accomplish well.

For more depth and detail, try these resources:

Col, N.F. 2005. Challenges in translating research into practice. *Journal of Women's Health* 14: 87–96.

Cullen, L., J. Greiner, J. Greiner, C. Bombei, and L. Comried. 2005. Excellence in evidence-based practice: organizational and unit exemplars. *Critical Care Nursing Clinics of North America* 17: 127–42.

Dean-Baar, S., and K. Pakieser-Reed. 2004. Closing the gap between research and clinical practice. *Topics in Stroke Rehabilitation* 11: 60–8.

Julian, D.C. 2005. Translation of clinical trials into clinical practice. *Journal of Internal Medicine Supplement* 742, 257: 12–20.

Klardie, K.A., J. Johnson, M.A. McNaughton, and W. Meyers. 2005. Integrating the principles of evidence-based practice into clinical practice. *Journal of the American Academy of Nurse Practitioners.* 16: 98, 100–2, 104–5.

Melnyk, B. and E. Fineout-Overholt. 2004. *Evidence-Based Practice in Nursing and Healthcare: A Guide to Best Practice*. Philadelphia: Lippincott, Williams and Wilkins.

Portney, L.G., and M.P. Watkins. 2000. *Foundations of Clinical Research: Applications to Practice,* 2nd ed. Upper Saddle River, NJ: Prentice Hall.

Shojania, K., and J. Grimshaw. 2005. Evidence-based quality improvement: The state of the science. *Health Affairs* 24: 138–53.

SUMMARY

Bedside scientists participate in a variety of ways in applied clinical research projects. They may be informed consumers of research and involved in research activities, participants on a team, or managers of research projects. Research is a necessary part of evidence-based practice and serves as the scientific basis for clinical care. A basis in research is a characteristic of a profession and enables the clinician to be accountable to patients.

Quality care is based on research, and many quality studies are very similar to practice-based research studies. Practice-based research is best carried out by a team, which involves developing collegial relationships. The team approach helps make research doable and improves the research itself through the availability of multiple perspectives. Understanding and using research in clinical practice are essential skills for the effective clinician.

CHAPTER 2

A Step-by-Step Guide
to Bedside Science Projects

In this chapter, you will learn to

- Use the steps of the research process to evaluate a research study
- Decide whether a systematic review or a focused research study is appropriate for a clinical question
- Participate as a team member in the design of a practice-based research project

*You frequently hear the terms **evidence-based medicine**, **evidence-based management**, and the term that applies to all disciplines, **evidence-based practice**. Today's goal is to have most, if not all, of what we do based on evidence—the best evidence, to be exact. Although a lot is heard about the concept, however, it seems like a tremendous amount of work to make it a reality.*

As a pharmacist, you regularly read and apply what you have read in professional journals. You feel fortunate, for most medications that eventually make it to practice are supported by one or more large, well-done, randomized controlled trials. You are, however, aware that evidence does not support many issues that surround medication delivery. It could be as simple as the use of a certain medication in the pediatric population or other vulnerable populations, or it could be the complex problems of medication adherence or avoidance of errors. You tackle the issue of medication reconciliation or the process of matching a patient's inpatient medications with those taken at home. You find a well-done, multisite study reported in a highly respected, peer-reviewed journal. The goal of the study was to understand the magnitude of the medication reconciliation issue in hospitals. The study was not a true randomized trial, however, because no control group existed. Rather, this was a descriptive study of an intervention in which all of the newly admitted patients had their medications reviewed by a pharmacist within the first 24 hours. The pharmacist checked to see whether their at-home medications were reconciled with their inpatient medications. Medication allergies and interactions were noted and dealt with. It was a great study, but in your environment you do not have the resources to commit a pharmacist full-time to this system. You look at some other alternatives. Several other studies supported the use of a "medication nurse" to do something similar, but still no comparison group was used. This might be an intervention your hospital could try: an advanced practice nurse/pharmacist team that made medication rounds on all new patients, consulting each other as needed. You think you can build a strong case and that the change would be worth it if you can find objective evidence of its effectiveness in avoiding medication interactions and errors. Perhaps you could measure where you are now—try your idea for a while and then see how you have fared? You would then have the evidence that you need to decide whether the investment is worth it without committing permanent resources. Your idea is turning into a research study. Simultaneously, you are going to need some help to do this right.

Practice supported by evidence is the goal for clinicians; achieving that goal remains a challenge. Connecting evidence to practice is valuable and can be done by bedside scientists. However, there is a special science to connecting evidence to practice. Like the skill that it takes to create a research project, finding the evidence to support a practice or to change practice is a structured and organized process.

Using methods that trial lawyers use in building a case, clinicians use the "best available evidence" from the literature, their clinical expertise, and consideration of their patient's values to build a case for a given clinical practice. Functioning much as a judge and jury, the evidence-based practitioner must critically evaluate and summarize the evidence and decide on a verdict. For the clinician, that verdict is the best demonstrated practice.

The process is one that requires knowledge about the research process so that studies can be read critically, followed by synthesis of the best findings into a single guideline. In most cases, the literature will provide most of the evidence you need. In some cases, however, you may need to conduct a focused study yourself to find out how a practice works with your patients in your setting or to fill a gap in the existing knowledge. Regardless, the process is systematic and rigorous and involves a step-by-step approach that focuses on evidence rather than anecdotes.

A systematic review of the research or a practice-based research study begins with a compelling clinical question. Some studies focus on life and death matters; others are related to comfort or satisfaction or performance-improvement issues. Your best studies will start with a question that you are passionate to answer. Regardless, the clinical question will drive the rest of the decisions you make and will eventually lead you to the ways you can improve outcomes for your patients. Whether you plan a systematic review or a practice-based research study, this is where the process begins.

STEP 1: DEFINE A RESEARCH QUESTION

After you identify a pressing matter or topic to study further, you will then need to frame it into a question, preferably a single question. The research question is about finding the right focus so that it is clear why this subject is important to study. Who are the people that interest you? What intervention will you use, and where and when will it be applied? Exactly how will you measure the effects of the intervention?

Let us return to our pharmacist's idea of seeing whether using nurse/pharmacists teams to accomplish medication reconciliation is effective. The question might be this: "Can using a nurse/pharmacist team to do medication reconciliation within the first 24 hours of a medical–surgical patient's admission decrease medication interactions?" In this case, the "who" is the medical–surgical patient. The "what" is the use of a nurse/pharmacist team for medication reconciliation. The "when" is during the first 24 hours, and the "how" is the measurement of medication interactions before and after the intervention.

You may wonder whether a research question is different from a question for a systematic review of the literature. The primary difference is that one ends up as an original research study, and the other ends up as an evaluation of the existing research. Both are research studies. Research and the systematic reviews that support evidence-based practice are often referred to as two separate processes when in fact they have a great deal of overlap. In fact, doing a systematic review requires that you have a strong understanding of research methods so that you can critically read and synthesize the best available evidence.

Spend time making sure that your research question is clear and focused, regardless of the method that will be used to answer it. The question leads you to your next step in the process: review of the literature.

STEP 2: SCAN THE LITERATURE

As you focus your question and build a case for practice, begin with a thorough search of the existing literature on your topic of interest. There are several ways to start. First, *search for an existing guideline* that is based on evidence. If guidelines do exist, they may be found at www.guidelines.gov, through your professional organization, or in a journal article listed in Ovid, Medline, or CINAHL. If no guideline can be found, *consider conducting a systematic review*, which is done exactly as its name implies—systematically. It is a method to evaluate the effectiveness of an intervention by identifying literature on the topic of interest, appraising that literature as evidence, and then synthesizing the findings into a report that encourages application of the findings to practice. It may happen that there is very little literature support for your question or that the evidence that does exist is based on weak studies. You may be unable to find studies that apply to your population and setting, or you may simply find no studies that focus on your specific question. In these cases, you may decide to *design a practice-based study to answer a focused research question.* If no evidence exists, you may need to design and carry out a research study as described in subsequent chapters of this book. It is possible, however, that evidence may exist for certain aspects of your question, and you just need to fill in the gaps. You have the option to build on the existing evidence, to replicate a study on your specific population, or to design a focused study to answer only part of the question.

For our pharmacist researcher, plenty of evidence shows that a patient's allergy or his or her at-home medications can result in adverse reactions, medication errors, or ineffective plans of care. However, no definitive guidelines exist for *how* medication reconciliation is accomplished. The descriptive studies are a good starting point but will not convince your administrator to invest in additional staff. To provide that evidence, you will need to look at what other organizations have done, find as many guidelines as you can, and build on the evidence that does exist. Clearly, you will need to develop and evaluate a method that works in your specific organization—this means a study focused on your nurse/pharmacist team idea that will provide the empirical evidence that you need to decide whether it works. The pharmacist will need more than an idea and motivation to see it through, however. A practice-based research study requires the help of many highly skilled people for effective design, data collection, and analysis. This will mean that resources will be needed—

perhaps financial and most certainly an investment of time—and thus, it is imperative that organizational commitment is sought and gained early in any bedside science project.

STEP 3: SOLICIT ORGANIZATIONAL COMMITMENT AND RESOURCES

Organizational commitment and the provision of resources are vital components of any study. Although commitment and resources do not assure that your study will be completed, a lack of them virtually guarantees failure. Even if the study involves only one clinical unit, it is crucial that you engage others

---

From the Mouths of Bedside Scientists: How Clinicians Talk About the Steps of Research

What are some do's and don'ts of research?

Oh—that is easy! You should *never* rush into doing a research study just to submit an abstract to a meeting that you want to attend. I did that once and will never do it again. I was not well focused, and my study was not as well designed as it could have been. I missed some important, recent studies that could have given me better direction in terms of my design. In fact, when I presented the results at a national critical care meeting, several experienced researchers shot them down. All I could do was thank them and go back to do a better study. Now, when I work with residents, I share this story as a warning. Your study puts your reputation on the line, and it should be the absolute best study to answer your question.

What step in the research process have you overlooked in the past?

I would have to say the literature search. Students and an assistant helped with a literature search, but I had to wade through lots of irrelevant studies and still missed several important studies. I never realized how much I could learn from the literature! I had a preconceived idea of what I wanted to study, but it turns out that I should have started with a more open mind . . . and better search terms.

I would always involve someone with statistical expertise at the beginning of my project. I waited until I was ready to have my data analyzed, and it turns out I had missed collecting some simple but important information. I ended up having to spend 2 days going back through charts to collect the additional information I needed.

to either give their blessing to do the study, provide input into design, or participate in data collection. It is best when those who will be affected by the study have representation on the investigative team.

Our pharmacist will need substantial organizational commitment for the medication reconciliation study. Nurse executives will need to provide an advanced practice nurse for the pilot team. The administrator in charge of the pharmacy will need to agree to the study and allocate resources for time, materials, and staffing. Salaries will need to be paid. Communications will have to be designed to let the team know when a new admission has arrived. Procedures will need to be developed to guide the medication reconciliation process; additional policies will guide the actions the nurse or pharmacist will take when a problem is found. Measures will need to be found for the expected outcomes, and information technology support will be needed to retrieve the data. Many departments will be affected by the pilot, and they will need time for thoughtful consideration of the project. Medical staff will need information about the pilot process and what it means for them and their patients. Their support in particular will be needed for the success of this project.

This step of identifying key stakeholders and gaining their support is particularly important if the study impacts hospital-wide care and requires substantial resources. Your two main needs will be research expertise and time. After you have a commitment from the right people to provide the support and resources for your study, the specifics of your research design must be identified. Your planning phase will require time for a review, critique, and summary of the evidence, followed by a thoughtful definition of your study methods and procedures.

STEP 4: DESIGN THE REVIEW OR STUDY WITH CAREFUL ATTENTION TO STUDY METHODS AND PROCEDURES

Your question will drive the review of the literature; your study design will be guided by what you found in the literature as well as by your specific question. The review of the evidence is really a study in itself. It is not about getting every possible piece of evidence on a topic. It is about getting focused evidence that both supports and opposes the premise of your research question and critically building a case for a specific clinical practice. In a sense, a systematic review of the literature is where your study begins. It will help guide you toward the best way to choose your study design to answer the research question that you have written.

If an intervention is evaluated, the focus is whether there is a difference in the group that received the intervention and whether the effects of the intervention can be isolated from all other effects. This requires an experimental

Hitting the Stacks

Lemstra, Stewart, and Olszynski (2002) demonstrated all of the steps in the clinical research process in their study of a multidisciplinary approach to the treatment of migraine:

Objective: To test the effectiveness of a multidisciplinary management program for migraine treatment in a group, low-cost, nonclinical setting.

Design: A prospective, randomized, clinical trial.

Methods: Eighty men and women were randomly assigned to one of two groups. The intervention group consisted of a neurologist and physical therapist intake and discharge, 18 group-supervised exercise therapy sessions, two group stress-management and relaxation-therapy lectures, one group dietary lecture, and two massage therapy sessions. The control group consisted of standard care with the patient's family physician. Outcomes were measured at the end of the 6-week intervention and at a 3-month follow-up.

Results: Forty one of 44 patients from the intervention group and all 36 patients from the control group completed the study. There were no statistically significant differences between the two groups before intervention. . . . Analysis revealed that the intervention group experienced statistically significant changes in self-perceived pain frequency ($p = 0.000$), pain intensity ($p = 0.001$), pain duration ($p = 0.000$), functional status ($p = 0.000$), quality of life ($p = 0.000$), health status ($p = 0.000$), pain-related disability ($p = 0.000$), and depression ($p = 0.000$). . . . There were no statistically significant changes in medication use or work status.

Conclusions: Positive health related outcomes in migraine can be obtained with a low-cost, group, multidisciplinary intervention in a community-based, nonclinical setting.

(Source: Lemstra, M., B. Stewart, and W. Olszynski. 2002. Effectiveness of multidisciplinary intervention in the treatment of migraine: A randomized clinical trial. *Headache* 42: 845–54.)

design. On the other hand, if the goal is a more thorough understanding of a specific topic, a descriptive study may be most appropriate and reasonable to accomplish. Some of the study designs that can be chosen are as follows:

- Randomized controlled trial: Individuals are randomly assigned to an intervention group or a control group, and differences between them are measured.

- Quasiexperimental designs: Comparison groups are used that are selected other than randomly.
- Cohort study: Different groups are followed over time.
- Predictive study: Groups of variables are tested to determine if an outcome can be predicted.
- Case/control study: Subjects with a risk factor are compared with subjects who do not have the risk factor to determine differences.
- Descriptive study: Objective or survey-based information is collected about specific individuals or groups.
- Qualitative studies: Observation and interaction are used to gather subjective information directly from subjects.

Detail as much about the study as you can before starting; nothing about the study methods should be left to chance. It is crucial to have a clear, thoughtful, well-written plan. If the plan is for a systematic review, provide specific detail about search terms, the study populations of interest, the kinds of studies that will be reviewed, and how the studies will be evaluated. If the plan is for a focused research study, determine the population of interest, the sampling strategy, the data collection process, and the analytic plan.

Our pharmacist successfully gained organizational support for the study and recruited a team to help with the research design. The intervention was specified, and assignments were made to write clear and thorough procedures for the nurse/pharmacist team intervention. Although the team wanted to include every new admission in the study, there would clearly be insufficient time and staff to accomplish that goal. An effective way to represent the entire population with a smaller, more accessible group was needed to make the study doable. The team decided that they could intervene with 20% of new admissions with the resources available. It was decided to compare the rate of drug interactions for the 20% that would receive the intervention with the rate for the 80% who would not. A sampling strategy was needed to gain efficiency while assuring the results would be valid and broadly applicable.

STEP 5: DETERMINE A SAMPLING STRATEGY

How many individuals you choose from your target population and the when, where, and how of your sampling plan need careful thought. Generalization of your study results will depend to a large extent on your sampling strategy. The sampling strategy includes how subjects are selected as well as how many subjects are needed.

A key point is that any element of randomness—either random selection or random assignment to groups—gives you the best ability to say that any differences you see happened because of the intervention and not from chance alone.

Strengthen Your Practice-Based Research Projects

Conducting research in a practice setting presents challenges for even the most seasoned researcher. Practice-based projects involve issues of organizational approval, subject recruitment, procedural control, and data collection that may be difficult to overcome. That does not mean, however, that practice-based research cannot be accomplished—and accomplished well.

- Accept the fact that practice-based research is messy and that you will not be able to have as much control over the research process as you might in a laboratory setting. Control what you can, and do not obsess over the things you cannot.

- Be systematic with your approach. Use the steps in this chapter in the right order, and carefully consider each design decision.

- If you cannot control a threat to validity (e.g., historical events), then move on and account for it in your write-up. As long as you are honest about what you could and could not control, your study will still be strong.

- Discuss your ideas with others, and consider their ideas with an open mind. Be creative in the way that you control validity in the applied setting. Get advice from experts within your organization or at local universities.

- Contact researchers who have done work similar to yours. You will be surprised at how easily you can get a researcher to talk about their work—most researchers are passionate about their subject and are willing to share procedures, ideas, and even instrumentation. Be considerate of their time, however, and use e-mail instead of the telephone for the researcher's convenience.

- Do not focus on resources that you do not have, but instead, capitalize on those you do. Substantial statistical analysis can be completed on Excel, for example. Under "tools" and then "add-ins," a statistical analysis package is available that you can turn on in any version of this common spreadsheet. The package will generate random numbers for sampling, calculate correlation coefficients and regression, and conduct a range of hypothesis tests, including t-tests, f-tests, and one-way analysis of variance.

- Use secondary data whenever possible. Secondary data—data that have already been collected—are easier to use and are more efficient to access.

- Do not assume that your organization has no research resources because you do not have a formal research department. Often there are people in the quality department, information technology, medical staff, or marketing unit that understand research concepts and can provide advice. Advance practice nurses, pharmacists, physical therapists, nutritionists, and a range of other professionals may also be able to provide input for your study. Do not overlook the medical librarian as a valuable source of help in finding literature for your study.

Randomness means that the sample will be representative of the larger population and supports generalization to broader groups. Random assignment does not need to be complicated—the flip of a coin or the roll of a die is sufficient. Without random sampling, however, the potential for selection bias exists. One group could have younger patients who are less likely to have multiple medications. The experimental group might have older patients or patients with chronic diseases that may require multiple medications. With random sampling or random assignment, groups should have similar characteristics.

A second key point is that the size of the sample should be determined through power analysis. Power analysis is a calculation based on the expected characteristics of the population, the number of variables to be analyzed, the type of statistical tests to be used, and the amount of certainty needed. A sample with sufficient power is one that is large enough to detect differences if they exist.

Our pharmacist-led research team decided that random sampling would be used to identify patients for baseline measurement. When admitting a new patient, the admissions clerks would roll a die. If the die landed on five, the team would be notified of the admission, and the patient would get a medication reconciliation consult after the specified procedures. Although one of six was not exactly 20%, it would be close. If the roll of the die resulted in any other number, the patient would receive standard medication management. The indicators would be recorded for all subjects so that they could be compared later. The team members consulted a statistician who calculated a power analysis; they knew they needed at least 120 subjects to draw definitive conclusions. With a sampling strategy and a design, the team was ready to begin the experiment.

STEP 6: COLLECT AND ANALYZE THE DATA

After the experiment begins, the intervention must be carried out carefully and consistently as specified in the study plan. Data are collected exactly as planned for every subject—experimental or control—according to protocols. Any departure from the plan could provide alternative explanations for your results. For example, using untrained personnel to provide the medication reconciliation, or measuring outcomes differently in the experimental group than in the control group, might result in differences that are due to something other than the intervention. The choice of an analytic test for the data is also an important issue. The data analysis is driven by the nature of the research question, the level of measurement, the sampling strategy, and the resources available.

Our pharmacist's study got off to a rocky start. Admissions clerks were inconsistent in rolling the die; referrals did not always make it to the team. Sometimes both the nurse and the pharmacist made a consult, and at other times,

> ## For more depth and detail, try these resources:
>
> Boissel, J. 2005. Planning of clinical trials. *Journal of Internal Medicine Supplement* 742, 257: 36–48.
>
> Creswell, J.W. 2003. *Research Design: Qualitative, Quantitative, and Mixed Methods,* 2nd ed. Thousand Oaks, CA: Sage Publications.
>
> Hudson, K. 2005. From research to practice on the Magnet pathway. *Nursing Management* 36: 33–8.
>
> Hulley, S.B., S.R. Cummings, W.S. Browner, D. Grady, N. Hearst, and T.B. Newman. 2001. *Designing Clinical Research*, 2nd ed. Philadelphia: Lippincott, Williams, and Wilkins.
>
> Melnyk, B., and E. Fineout-Overholt. 2004. *Evidence-Based Practice in Nursing and Healthcare: A Guide to Best Practice.* Philadelphia: Lippincott, Williams and Wilkins.
>
> Portney, L.G., and M.P. Watkins. 2000. *Foundations of Clinical Research: Applications to Practice,* 2nd ed. Upper Saddle River, NJ: Prentice Hall.

neither of them did. It was clear that the initial part of the experiment would be unusable, other than to find and fix the glitches in the experiment. The team decided to continue the experiment for a month as a pilot and then reconvene and determine next steps. After the pilot month, however, the experiment started clicking. Referrals were coming in and communications were clearing up. Patients were being seen, and data were being captured. The team decided that it was time for a full-blown attempt to get the 120 subjects they needed.

Two months later, it was time for analysis. The team had 116 subjects in their experimental group and about five times that in their control group. Workload for everyone on the team had crept back up, and few resources were left for more data collection. The statistician was confident that enough data were available for an accurate analysis. After all of their work, the team members felt exhausted but waited excitedly for the results of their work. They were ready to find out whether the test would result in a change in practice that would improve the care of their patients.

STEP 7: APPLICATION AND COMMUNICATION

The end of a study is the culmination of a lot of hard work. It is, however, just the beginning of even harder work: making a change in practice. Although this sounds simple, even the easiest change requires careful thought, a way to evaluate compliance and then to evaluate the impact of the change on your population.

Communication throughout every stage of the practice change is critical and helps assure buy-in at all levels. Begin by sharing the evidence for the change with staff and other colleagues. Discuss the implementation plan, and get feedback from those who will be affected. Share what you find as implementation progresses and as you evaluate the impact of and compliance with the change. In an overall way, communication is part of the intervention.

A practice change is usually carried out in limited fashion first, as a pilot. Then, if successful, the change is expanded to more units. It is important to set up and evaluate the practice change using sound research methods. Continuous measurement will assure that the intervention is applied in practice as it was designed and that outcomes achieved during the experiment are maintained.

Back to our medication reconciliation research team—they are ecstatic to determine that the subjects in the experimental group demonstrated superior outcomes to those receiving the standard approach. The findings are communicated to leadership groups, and additional staffing hours are assigned to implement the service on a limited number of units. Expansion of the service is approved as time progresses, and the service is streamlined. The team begins discussing the presentation of their findings at conferences and the potential for a publication. There is a clear sense of accomplishment and of making a contribution to the organization and to health care in general.

SUMMARY

Clinical research for bedside scientists starts with a compelling research question that will drive the remainder of the process. Sometimes a clinical question can be answered with a literature review. The development of a practice guideline requires a systematic review process, one that has guidelines similar to the design of a research study. When a lack of available, applicable, or appropriate research exists, focused studies may be needed. When designing a bedside science project, organizational commitment and resources are needed early in the process. After support is available, a collaborative research team can best make decisions about study design, sampling strategy, data collection, analysis, and application. Communication is a critical element of the implementation plan, and demonstration pilots can be an effective way to accomplish implementation.

Final communication to the larger profession through conferences and publication is the last step in transferring knowledge from limited experiments to a broader audience. Although a challenging undertaking, this is a valuable way to contribute to science. The long, arduous process of initiating a practice change begins, and the contribution of an evidence-based practice emerges.

Concepts in Action

Doing a study to help you better understand why something unusual is happening to your patients can give you the data you need to improve patient care. The example that follows shows how a study was carefully designed and implemented to address a unit concern. This became a research question that eventually created some important practice changes. As you read this scenario, consider how you might use a bedside science project to address patient care issues in your own setting.

What was the question studied in this bedside science project?

Which fall risk characteristics are more common in older, transitional (skilled) care patients who have nonserious falls when compared with those who do not fall?

Why was this research question important?

Falls in older patients are always a concern in an inpatient, transitional care setting because of the impact on length of stay and satisfaction with care. This unit had many processes in place to assess risk and prevent falls. Even so, the unit experienced a few nonserious falls every month, and over one 5-month period noticed a spike in the number of falls. Only one case was serious, requiring hip surgery, but any type of injury is significant to the patient who falls. Minor injuries included abrasions, contusions, lacerations, skin tears, and complaints of "soreness" or pain in areas affected by the fall. The nursing staff members were concerned because they knew that even a minor injury could cause discomfort, impact quality of life, and affect responsiveness to therapy. Usual causes were investigated, such as toileting needs, diagnosis type, or inadequate staffing, and no consistent cause was found. The unit staff decided to evaluate the rise in falls using research methods.

Who was involved on the research team?

The unit nurse director led the study and engaged a small team of colleagues, including a healthcare researcher, two physical therapists, two staff nurses, and a nurses' aide. Other health care professionals on the unit, including physicians, bedside nurses, and housekeeping were involved through unit discussions.

(continues)

Concepts in Action *(continued)*

What were the methods that were planned?

A systematic review was done to understand what factors were most associated with older patients who sustained a nonserious fall. The team designed a prospective study, using a case-control approach to compare characteristics of fallers and nonfallers. Patients were included in this study if they were admitted to a transitional (skilled) care unit and sustained a fall during a 1-year data collection period (cases) or were an age and gender-matched nonfaller admitted to the same unit during the same time period (controls).

The study team spent a significant amount of time creating and piloting a data collection form. Many unit staff members were asked for feedback on the data collection method, the content of questions, and the way to ask them. The staff was asked whether they believed the responses would answer the research question. The sampling method was straightforward, as the sample size was limited to the number of patients who fell during the year of their study.

Inclusion criteria for the study were essentially the criteria for admission to the unit. These included having a 3-day hospital stay within the previous 30 days; a demonstrated need for skilled services, including nursing care and/or physical or occupational therapy; and a reasonable discharge plan. Most of the patients were admitted from a hospital unit and had a variety of medical–surgical problems, including stroke, major joint replacements, cancer, surgical wounds, and cardiac, pulmonary, or neurologic exacerbations.

In the case group, falls were categorized into the type of fall. First, "fall" was defined as an event in which the resident unintentionally came to rest on the ground or the floor regardless of subsequent injury. A "witnessed" fall was one in which hospital staff observed the resident in the act of falling. If staff were close enough to intervene, the fall was described as an "assist to the floor," regardless of any injury as a result of the fall. Controls were residents admitted to the unit during the same time period and were matched to the cases for age and gender.

The team planned to review each fall within 72 hours of the occurrence. Fall-specific data were to be collected on those who fell, including characteristics of the fall, risk factors at the time of the fall, and interventions in place to prevent the fall. Data from cases and controls included intervention plans and descriptive data. The data collection plan appears in Table 2-1.

(continues)

Table 2-1   Data Collection for Fall Risk Study

Category of Data	Data Element	Collected For
Data related to the fall	Time of fall Day of fall Subjective fall risk Witnessed or unwitnessed Any injury as a result of the fall Type of fall	Cases (residents who fell)
Potential fall risks	Footwear at time of fall Mental status IV therapy Environmental factors (e.g., wet floors, clutter) Medications in the 24 hours prior to the fall	Cases
Fall risk interventions	Use of a bed/chair alarm or nurse no-tification system Patient's use of call bell immediately before the fall Presence of staff to intervene or lower the resident to the floor Presence of a nursing care plan iden-tifying the patient as a high fall risk Presence of a bed/chair/alarm or nurse notification system Use of an ambulation device Presence of a toileting plan	Cases Cases and controls
Descriptive data	Gender Age Date of admission to the unit Admitting diagnosis History of falls Visual impairment Presence of neuropathy Mobility impairment Categories of medications	Cases and controls

Concepts in Action *(continued)*

What challenges were faced?

After data collection was begun, the number of falls decreased. This was likely due to the Hawthorne effect, as staff awareness was heightened. A new fall risk-assessment tool was found about halfway through the study period and was considered for implementation because of its ability to predict the likelihood of a fall. This tool took into consideration most of the factors already being considered by this project. It introduced a threat to validity because unit procedures changed during the study.

A limitation of this project was that fallers (cases) were compared with nonfallers (controls), and thus, several issues specifically related to falling could only be described in the faller group. This is a general weakness of the case-control design and not just this specific study. Retrospective review reveals information on cases that cannot be collected on controls simply because they do not experience the phenomenon under study. Numbers of falls per month were low—which was a good thing—but they were insufficient to enable analysis of trends.

During initial pilot analysis for design of the study, the team noticed that during 3 high-fall months, many falls occurred during very early morning (between 4 a.m. and 6 a.m.). Before the study began, the unit implemented changes that addressed this issue, specifically nurse aide rounds during this time period each morning. The aides also reassured patients the night before that they could call staff in the early morning hours because several patients reported they did not want to "disturb" the nurse at that hour of the morning. This falls into the category of historical threats to internal validity or alternative explanations for findings that are due to process changes midway through the study.

After data collection and analysis were complete, the team members identified data that they would have liked to consider. It is not unusual that gaps in the data collection plan are found during analysis and write-up, and this study was no exception. The team identified that future studies should also collect data about additional staffing issues and family presence.

How were the results of the study used?

Characteristics of the study population were carefully reviewed, and areas for improvement were identified and then classified as "quick fixes" or "longer term fixes."

Concepts in Action *(continued)*

The 82 study cases and 82 control patients were similar in age and gender to usual patients on this unit, with most in their late 70s and around two thirds being women. When comparing the fallers and their matched controls, some important findings were revealed. Fallers were more likely to have a mobility impairment (87.8%, n = 72, p < 0.0001) and were less likely to have been regularly using an ambulatory device than nonfallers (p < 0.0001). Only 19 were actually using an ambulatory device (e.g., cane, walker, or quad cane) at the time of the fall. Physical therapy, nursing staff, and the resident's family members were notified of this finding, and special precautions were put in place. These included early intensive physical therapy and training in use of ambulatory and other assistive devices.

Special attention was given to visual issues. Fallers were more likely to have some type of visual impairment (42.8%, n = 35, p = 0.007), including a history of visual problems, such as cataracts, glaucoma, or the need for corrective lenses. Eleven of the fallers were actually wearing glasses at the time of their fall, although specific information about their eyeglasses, such as correctness of the prescription, was not available.

Of patients who fell, 34% of the falls occurred on admission through the first 72 hours, and a whopping 46.3% occurred between days 4 to 14. The remaining 19.1% sustained a fall between day 15 and day 60. Because 54.9% of patients who fell had a previous history of falls within the last 90 days, these patients were identified as high risk. Fall prevention plans were frequently assessed during the first 14 days after a resident's admission as a result of the study findings.

The *lack* of some differences between the groups was almost as surprising as the differences. Patients with a history of osteoporosis did not experience more falls than those without osteoporosis. Only 12 of the residents (14.6%) with a history of osteoporosis fell during the study period; however, almost as many did not fall, and the difference was not significant. Although confusion is frequently identified as a fall risk, only 29 (35.4%) of the fallers were confused at time of their fall and this percentage was not different than nonfallers. Neuropathy did not prove to be an indicator of fall risk, as only three (3.7%) had this as a primary or secondary diagnosis at the time of the fall. Anticoagulation therapy has been cited as a fall risk factor because of the increased risk of injury, but it was not significantly different in this sample.

(continues)

Concepts in Action *(continued)*

There was an association between use of several medications within 24 hours of the fall and a subsequent fall and included the use of psychotropic medications ($p < 0.001$) and use of one or more antihypertensive medications ($p < 0.0001$).

Many of the falls were unwitnessed ($n = 60$, 73%), and of the 22 falls that were witnessed, the staff was able to intervene and "assist to the floor" 11 times. It is not known from these data whether staff interventions were positively correlated to injury prevention in this group. Of residents who fell, 73 (89%) did not use the nurse call system to seek assistance before the fall, although these systems were in place in all rooms. It was unknown how frequently the nonfallers used the call system.

The majority of falls (66, 80.5%) occurred in the resident's room near the bed. Only 8 falls (9.75%) occurred in the bathroom. The remaining falls occurred in other areas such as the unit corridor (hallway), shower room, or the therapy department. There did not appear to be problems with clutter, wet floor, or inadequate footwear that contributed to the falls.

This team identified a problem, designed a realistic study to evaluate the problem, and made changes based on data analysis. The fall rate for both noninjury and injury falls continued to decrease throughout the duration of the project.

How were the study's results communicated internally and to larger audiences?

The results were presented at a hospital research day and at several national nursing conferences. Plans are currently underway to publish the results in a peer-reviewed journal.

Part II

Building a Foundation for a Bedside Science Project

CHAPTER 3

Focus the Research Question

In this chapter, you will learn to
• Identify some sources of research questions in clinical practice • Translate a clinical problem into a research question • Focus and refine a research question with all of the necessary elements • Describe the link between the research question and the study design • Turn a research question into a testable hypothesis

You have been interested in the topic of patient satisfaction but are not sure how to turn your idea into a research question. You talk to your colleagues and your family about the topic, and start observing how people treat you when you are at a store or checking in to a hotel. You begin to pay attention to your feelings about the way people treat you and how your mood might affect how you feel about the way people are treating you. Many things go into your own "feelings" of satisfaction. Thus, you decide to begin searching the literature on this topic. The Google search engine gets 84,600,000 hits. Because this seems to be too much, you do a quick search in Ovid MEDLINE, getting 66,333 articles. This question will definitely need to be focused. You decide to look at satisfaction with medical care. Now 41,760 abstracts need to be reviewed. You realize that you will need to be really specific.

Think back to why you even thought about studying satisfaction in the first place: your unit gets rated on how satisfied the patients are with their care, but you have never been sure about how you can affect the satisfaction level. Your unit is pediatric intensive care, and thus, the person actually rating your care is one or both parents or a legal guardian. You will now need to look at the issue of parental satisfaction with a critically ill child's care. Then you begin thinking about what things affect "care." Many individuals care for the critically ill child during their stay on your unit. Because you are a clinician on a multidisciplinary team that takes care of critically ill children, you decide to focus on one aspect of care that all disciplines must do: communication with parents. Now the topic is more focused. You begin reading articles about clinician communication with parents while their child is in intensive care and how this affects the parents' response. Communication is a well-defined problem with many aspects to study: What information is shared? How often should it be shared? How should it be shared? Clearly you need a specific, focused research question if your study is to be doable and still address the problem identified.

Every research question begins with an idea, a thought, a hunch, an uncertainty, or an observation that gave you pause and made you wonder "what if?" As a clinician, you often tuck away the idea, thinking about it now and then. Much later at a conference or in a journal article you may find that someone studied the question you are interested in. As you hear or read about their methods, however, you realize that they did not specifically address the question you had or they addressed it in a way that is not applicable to your environment. Thus, you begin exploring the question further and consider doing your own study. This illustrates one common way that research questions are discovered and translated into real studies. This chapter helps you understand the concept of the focused research question, and the way it gives direction for most study elements.

The most important component of a study is the research question. It defines your study. Everything that follows the question reflects how well you shape your research question.

WHERE TO FIND RESEARCH PROBLEMS

Challenges exist in going from a clinical problem to a researchable question. As healthcare professionals, we are generally quite good at identifying problems and looking for solutions to them. Identifying a problem motivates us to find a solution to the problem. Asking good questions helps to identify solutions. Finding empirical evidence that a solution effectively addresses a problem is an outcome of good research.

Some problems and the associated questions are specific to one patient or to a specific type of patient population. Some relate to the healthcare environment in which care is provided. Others might relate to how we are feeling or to discovering how our patients feel. Research problems may also come from sources other than patient care and the environment. Reading professional journal articles, listening to conference presentations, and reading unit reports may also lead to researchable problems. Good research questions come from any source and arise from clinical curiosity combined with a healthy skepticism about "the way things have always been done."

Good sources of researchable questions may start out as quality-improvement studies. Quality data may point to problems with processes on the unit or with certain kinds of patients, diagnoses, or procedures.

The best research questions come from issues or problems that are fascinating or that you are passionate about. Research takes effort, and continued enthusiasm about a project is rooted in your interest in making the situation better. Refining the research question will assure that your project is doable and will guide the development of your research design.

REFINE THE RESEARCH QUESTION

The way to refine a research question is similar to how a diagnosis or a patient problem statement is refined. What do you already know about the topic? What do you believe about it? Refining is similar to focusing a microscope—as you focus more tightly, the details become clear. You will go from general to more specific as you progress to the final version of your question.

Begin by defining the "who, what, when, where, and how" aspects of your question. Who is the identified population of interest? What intervention do you think will be effective in solving the problem? What will you measure to determine whether it is effective? When, where, and how will you measure the outcome?

Next, briefly search the available literature to find out what is already known about the problem. The literature may also help to focus your question, or it may provide you with studies you can replicate. You may find an example of a question that needs only minor revisions to work for your study. Conversely, very little might be known about the topic, in which case further study is warranted.

Hitting the Stacks

Jones, Marini, and Slate (2005) had several questions they wanted to address in their research about the differences in prevention practices between persons who had spinal cord injuries with rare pressure ulcers and those whose pressure ulcers were frequent. Instead of creating a single, complicated, compound question, they broke the question into four very specific questions. "We explored what behavioral management wellness strategies/habits persons with SCI [spinal cord injury] who rarely, if ever, sustain a pressure ulcer use in their daily lives and compared this group with those who have recurrent problems with pressure ulcers. Four research questions were posed:

1. Is there a differential effect in pressure ulcer prevention strategies for persons with SCI with healthy skin versus similarly injured persons with pressure ulcer problems?

2. Is there a differential effect in occurrence of pressure ulcers between those persons with SCI with healthy skin versus similarly injured persons with pressure ulcer problems when compared by demographic factors?

3. Is there a differential effect in occurrence of pressure ulcers between those persons with SCI with healthy skin versus similarly injured persons with pressure ulcer problems when compared by health and wellness behaviors?

4. Is there a differential effect in occurrence of pressure ulcers between those persons with SCI with healthy skin versus similarly injured persons with pressure ulcer problems when compared by disability-specific characteristics?"

Patel, Liebling, and Murphy (2003) also had more than one focus for their research on the effects of operative delivery on the success of breastfeeding. These authors stated their research questions as "aims," which is common verbiage for research questions funded by grants. "The aims of this study were twofold: the first was to compare the rates of exclusive breastfeeding at hospital discharge and at six weeks in women who had either instrumental vaginal delivery . . . or cesarean section at full cervical dilatation; and the second was to evaluate the effect of timing of discharge on breastfeeding rates."

Jones, M., I. Marini, and J. Slate. 2005. Prevention practice differences among persons with spinal cord injuries who rarely versus frequently sustain pressure ulcers. *Rehabilitation Counseling Bulletin* 48: 139–45.

Patel, R., R. Liebling, and D. Murphy. 2003. Effect of operative delivery in the second stage of labor on breastfeeding success. *Birth* 30: 255–60.

For example, if you are asking a question about an observed side effect of a particular drug, you can quickly look up all of the available information about the drug and its side effects to see whether your observation is truly unusual. Look at drug inserts, or do a quick literature search. If you do not find anything specific about the side effect, talk with colleagues to see whether they are noticing the same side effect when their patients take the drug. You might focus your question on a specific patient population that takes the drug and has the side effect, or you might want to compare patients with the side effect to patients without it.

Questions about processes of care are a little more difficult to study. Often, several questions need to be addressed. Medication errors are an example. Errors in medications may be the result of failed communication during crucial transition points in the continuum of care: admission, transfers between care settings, and discharge. In studying this problem, your research question might relate to communication issues involving hospital personnel at one or more of the crucial transition points or could focus on staffing issues, time management, skill level of staff, or any number of other possibilities. A challenge in studying processes is narrowing the study down to one aspect of the process so that the study is not unnecessarily complicated and is achievable.

As you continue the refinement process, critique your question continuously. The simple act of writing it down may help you focus and refine your question even better. Share it with your colleagues. Does it make sense? Is it logical? Is this question important for clinical care? Could there be practical benefits from this research? Are others interested who could help with your study?

THE ELEMENTS OF A GOOD QUESTION

Two guides are helpful in developing a good research question. One of them is described by the acronym FINER (Hulley & Cummings, 2001, p. 14) and refers to the following characteristics of a good question:

- **F**easible: adequate subjects, technical expertise, time, and money are available; the scope is narrowed enough for study.
- **I**nteresting: the question is interesting to the investigator.
- **N**ovel: the study confirms or refutes previous findings or provides new findings.
- **E**thical: the study cannot cause unacceptable risk to participants and does not invade privacy.
- **R**elevant: the question is relevant to scientific knowledge, clinical and health policy, or future research directions.

Another model gives guidance in the actual development of a question. The four elements represented by the PICO acronym outline the parts of a good

From the Mouths of Bedside Scientists: How Clinicians Talk About Research Questions

How has a question guided your research?

When I first got the idea of evaluating how parental anxiety impacted the way a physician treated a child, I was not sure how to design the study. This was an important topic to study because many of my physician and nurse colleagues have the "gut" feeling that anxious parents drive physicians to order more tests or treatments than they might otherwise do. We particularly noticed this in our bronchiolitis patients. When we got specific about what we wanted to study, the question ended up, "Does parental anxiety influence how a pediatrician takes care of a child with bronchiolitis, as evidenced by the number of tests ordered and length of stay?" To decide on a design, we had to look at the question carefully. Because we have clear guidelines for the treatment of bronchiolitis and we have this diagnosis on the unit frequently, I knew this study could be prospective. I also knew there needed to be some type of "blinding" so that the physicians would not know how parents were rating their anxiety level and be "influenced" by the study itself.

Where have your questions come from?

Our question—"Does foot massage in inpatient cancer patients reduce anxiety and improve satisfaction?"—came from both our clinical experience with cancer patients and from information we heard at a conference. On the unit, we noticed that if patients were anxious, we could use a standing order for antianxiety medication, but we could offer nothing else to the patient. When we heard how massage in cancer patients makes them feel more relaxed, we decided to explore the feasibility of doing it with our patients in our unit. We searched the literature on the topic, developed a multidisciplinary clinical research team, and spoke with several massage therapists to help refine our research question and design our study. We found that many different types of massage exist, and foot massage seemed to be a type that we could give to any cancer patient with minimal side effects.

Sometimes, the best ideas are found from the previous studies' failures. It is critical, as a researcher, to question everything and to explain the unknown, even if you feel that there are not any easy answers.

Ideas for good studies come from the inquisitive mind of a researcher. These ideas may be based on prior experiences, interests, or even dreams. The support system surrounding the research is what actually makes these ideas come to life.

question. Using preoperative education for short-stay patients undergoing prostatectomy as an example, a research question based on PICO might look as follows:

- **P**atient or problem: "In radical prostatectomy patients staying in the hospital one day after surgery . . ."
- **I**ntervention: ". . . does customized preoperative teaching . . ."
- **C**omparison intervention: ". . . compared with standard preoperative teaching . . ."
- **O**utcomes: ". . . lead to better pain control as measured by a visual analog scale?"

After your question is carefully defined, then the link to design elements often becomes obvious. If not, then you may need to continue getting more specific about the population, intervention, and outcomes. These three elements of the question provide guidance in the selection of a sample, the procedures that you will test, and the way that you will measure the results.

THE LINK BETWEEN QUESTIONS AND DESIGN

As you focus your research question, you will realize that how you ask the question will guide how you will answer the question. Your question will lead you to a sampling strategy (who is the patient population?), an intervention protocol (what treatment are you testing?), and the outcomes you will measure (how will you know its effect?). There are also direct links between the kind of words used in the question and the design that is used to answer it.

Descriptive Questions

Descriptive studies answer simple questions about what is happening in a defined population or situation. For example, the question "how many patients reporting high satisfaction with therapy had adequately controlled pain during their hospitalization?" can be answered by a descriptive design. Sometimes a descriptive study is called a *hypothesis-generating* study, contrasted with *hypothesis-testing* studies. Three general research questions are best answered with descriptive studies: (1) studies that investigate resource allocation, (2) studies that identify areas for further research, and (3) studies that provide informal diagnostic information.

Analytic Questions

Analytic studies relate one or more interventions to specific outcomes. For example, the questions "is it more effective to educate hip surgery patients

---

Strengthen Your Research Question

The most important part of the research process is getting the question right. How the problem is stated determines what measures will be used, what data will be collected, the kind of analysis that will be used, and the conclusions that can be drawn. It is worth the time, then, to consider carefully how this element of the research study is developed. A thoughtful process does not necessarily mean a complicated process, however. Here are some simple suggestions for creating strong research questions:

- Answer the "why" question first. With a solid understanding of the reason for the study, the specifics of the research question are easier to identify.

- Review the literature before you finalize the question. Do not hesitate to replicate the question of a research study that accomplishes the same goals that you have. It is flattering to a researcher—even those who are established and well known—to have their work replicated. Just be sure you give credit where credit is due.

- Focus, focus, focus. Refine your research question, mull it over for a bit, and then refine it again. The effort you spend to get the question just right will be worth it, as there will be less confusion later as to how to answer the question.

- Do not wait until your question is perfect to begin the design of your study. The question is, to some extent, a work in progress as you proceed with the specifics of your research. The question can—and likely will—be revised as new information, resources, and constraints come to light.

- Be sure to include the four major elements: Who is the population? What will be measured? How will it be measured? When will it be measured?

- Keep your research questions focused on these elements, but do not include more than one major concept per question. Compound questions are hard to study and make it harder to isolate the effects of a single variable. If you are sure you have to study more than one intervention or outcome, use multiple research questions instead of multiple parts of a single question.

---

about postop care with group education or practice visits?" and "is breast cancer associated with high fat intake?" are answered with quantitative analysis. The objective of an analytic study is to see whether a causal relationship exists between variables, and thus, the research question would reflect study of the effect of an intervention on one or more outcomes. Statistical procedures are used to see whether a relationship would likely have occurred by chance alone. Analytic studies usually compare two or more groups, such as comparing cases with a condition to controls without it (case-control design), randomized controlled clinical trials, and laboratory studies.

Analytic questions are not limited to prospective studies, however. Comparison studies—sometimes called contemporary comparison, causal comparison, or retrospective studies—investigate the differences between groups that are formed based on the presence or absence of a shared characteristic. A question that reflects studying two groups for similarities or differences in specified characteristics is answered with comparison studies. The question "do sedentary men over the age of 50 have heart attacks as frequently as sedentary women over the age of 50?" is answered with a comparison study. Comparison studies are needed when the research question is focused on a variable that cannot be practically or ethically manipulated, such as exposure to a risk factor or the diagnosis of a specific disease.

Questions that focus on associations or relationships are generally answered with correlation studies. Technically classified as descriptive studies, correlation studies focus on the relationships between two variables in the same population (e.g., height and weight) or between the same variable in two populations (e.g., height of fathers and sons.) Research questions focused on predicting one variable given the presence of another (e.g., can the height of the son be predicted if we know the height of the father?) are answered with a type of correlation study called a regression analysis.

Questions that are written in future tense will be answered with prospective studies. Interventions, data collection, and outcomes happen after subjects are enrolled. Examples of prospective studies are clinical trials and cohort studies. Prospective studies are indicated by research questions that focus on conditions that occur often with relatively short follow-up periods. These two criteria are necessary so that sufficient numbers of eligible individuals can be followed for a reasonable period of time.

If a research question is written in past tense, it will be a retrospective study. All events of interest have already occurred, and data are generated from records of the past (secondary data) or by asking subjects to recall events. Questions that focus on past relationships or the outcomes of events that have already occurred will be answered by retrospective study. Retrospective studies are less expensive than prospective studies and are often good starting points for exploratory research questions. Retrospective studies are far more effective when the research question involves a rare event, as patient records of rare events are generally available even when few subjects are available to recruit.

Analytic studies are logical for questions answered with numbers or with measurement. These quantitative studies involve testing research questions using statistical analysis. Although research questions are not directly testable with numbers, their transformed version—the hypothesis—is subject to numer-

---

Where to Look for Information About the Research Question or Hypothesis

- The research question may be explicitly stated in the research abstract but is commonly only implied by the title of the article, the purpose statement, or the objectives for the study.
- Ideally, the question is discussed at the beginning of the article, often at the end of the introduction. When it is stated early, it is followed by evidence from the literature review to support why this question is important to investigate further. It may be written as a statement instead of a question. If not at the beginning, look for the question at the end of the literature review.
- The null and alternate hypotheses are often found in the methods section where statistical methods are discussed, along with the rationale for the statistical tests used to test the hypotheses. Hypotheses are typically easy to find and are explicitly identified as such.
- Sometimes a separate section is created for a formal statement of the problem, the purpose of the study, and the research question. It may be labeled "Purpose," "Aims," or "Objectives." The research question may similarly have its own heading.
- If the researcher used any inferential statistical tests (which most quantitative studies do), then there were hypotheses, whether they are stated or not. Sometimes the reader is left to infer what the hypotheses were based on the tests that were reported.

---

ical analysis. It is therefore important to translate quantitative research questions into hypothesis statements that lend themselves to statistical analysis.

FROM QUESTION TO HYPOTHESIS

Just as the research question guides the design of a study, the hypothesis guides the statistical analysis. The way a hypothesis is written will determine what tests are run, what outcome is expected, and how conservative the results are. A hypothesis is a restatement of the research question in a form that can be analyzed statistically for significance. For example, the research question "can installation of new carpet trigger reactive airway disease in otherwise healthy adults?" can be rewritten as a hypothesis as "there is no association between the installation of new carpet and the onset of reactive airway disease in otherwise healthy adults." While stating there is "no expected relationship" might seem a counterintuitive way to start a research analysis, it is, in fact, the only way that statistical significance can be measured. Although we cannot ever be sure that a relationship *exists*, we can calculate the probability that it *does not*. Testing a null hypothesis in effect tells us *how much* uncertainty there is in our statistical conclusions, and thus, we can judge whether it is within an acceptable range.

Another Way to Look at It

Hypotheses can be confusing. Null hypotheses may seem particularly counterintuitive: why would a researcher start a study claiming that they will not find anything significant? The logic of hypothesis testing can be elusive, but it *is* based on solid reasoning. The first reason is purely statistical: hypotheses are statements that are directly testable with quantitative techniques, and research questions are not. The second reason is more philosophical. We cannot ever be *completely* sure that an outcome was caused *solely* by a treatment. We cannot directly test that a relationship is present. We can only estimate the chance that it is absent. Although we cannot prove an experiment worked, we can calculate the probability that the treatment worked purely by random chance.

Hopefully, most of us will never need a null hypothesis in its most common form—that of being charged with a crime. When someone is indicted for a crime, the relationship between the individual and the crime is stated as a null hypothesis. In other words, the accused is innocent until proven guilty. The initial assumption is that no relationship exists between the suspect and the crime. The prosecutor must show beyond a reasonable doubt—or beyond random chance—that the assumption of no relationship is wrong. If enough evidence is presented to convince 12 typical citizens that the assumption of innocence is wrong, then the jury will conclude that the relationship between the crime and the suspect is real.

Testing of a null hypothesis is similar to this process. The researcher starts the experiment with a statement that there is no relationship between the intervention and the outcome. If evidence is studied and there is not enough to convince the researcher that any relationship between the cause and the effect is real, then the initial idea of no relationship is supported. The null hypothesis is accepted, and no relationship is discovered. If, on the other hand, the majority of the evidence leads to a conclusion that the relationship does not happen by chance (usually less than 5% probability), then the researcher concludes that the null hypothesis must be wrong, and the treatment works. Although a null hypothesis may feel like a backward way to start a study, in reality, it raises the bar above random chance for drawing conclusions about the effectiveness of treatments.

Two aspects exist that make a good hypothesis: the statement of an expected relationship (or the lack of one) and an identified direction of interest. A null hypothesis states that *there is no difference between groups*, whereas an alternative hypothesis would *specify an expected difference between groups*. In either case, the relationship between variables is defined. A second consideration is directionality. A nondirectional hypothesis is one that means that the researcher is interested in a change in any direction—good or bad. In other words, a positive or negative association would be of interest. If we were testing a drug for hypertension, a nondirectional hypothesis would indicate that we were interested in the drug's effect in reducing blood pressure, but we would also be interested in whether it raised blood pressure. Sometimes called two-sided hypotheses, these are appropriate for exploratory research ques-

For more depth and detail, try these resources:

Findley, T.W. 1989. Research in physical medicine and rehabilitation: I: How to ask the question. *American Journal of Physical Medicine and Rehabilitation* 68: 26–31.

Greenblatt, M., G. Dickinson, and C. Simpson. 2004. Implementing the research question. *Knowledge Quest* 33: 75–6.

Hudson-Barr, D. 2005. From research idea to research question: The who, what, where, when, and why. *Journal for Specialists in Pediatric Nursing* 10: 90–2.

Law, R. 2004. From research topic to research question: A challenging process. *Nurse Researcher* 11: 54–66.

Leedy, P., and J. Ormrod. 2005. *Practical Research: Planning and Design*, 8th ed. Upper Saddle River, NJ: Pearson Merrill Prentice Hall.

Meadows, K. 2003. So you want to do research? 2: Developing the research question. *British Journal of Community Nursing* 8: 397–405.

Morgan, G., and R. Harmon. 2000. Research questions and hypotheses. *Journal of the American Academy of Child and Adolescent Psychiatry* 39: 251–4.

Morrison, J. 2002. Developing research questions in medical education: The science and the art. *Medical Education* 36: 596–8.

Portney, L., and M. Watkins. 2000. *Foundations of Clinical Research: Applications to Practice*, 2nd ed. Upper Saddle River, NJ: Prentice Hall Health.

Stone, P. 2002. Deciding upon and refining a research question. *Palliative Medicine* 16: 265–8.

tions or randomized trials of interventions. These are more rigorous tests than directional hypotheses.

Directional hypotheses, or one-sided tests, test only one direction of change. These are appropriate for research questions in which a great deal of literature or empirical support is available for an existing relationship. Directional hypothesis tests are more liberal than nondirectional ones.

SUMMARY

The clinical environment is a rich breeding ground for ideas that can become research questions. What interests you? What problems would you like to see solved? What are you curious about? What treatments are you skeptical about? Any of these questions could generate research ideas. When the purpose of a study is clearly focused, then the research question is carefully defined. Focus on *who* will be studied, *what* intervention will be used, and *how* the outcome will be measured.

The research question is the most critical element of a study. Careful construction of the research question is worth the time and effort, as it sets the stage for a clear and effective study design.

Concepts in Action

The design of any research project is driven by the specifics of the research question. Bedside scientists are well advised to spend time and thought on this critical part of the research process. In the following example, the research question was one that dictated an experimental design, as the question focused on the results of an experimental intervention. A question of this sort requires that we have a sample that represents the population well—and has an element of randomness—and that extraneous variables are controlled. This experiment used strict protocols, inclusion and exclusion criteria, and objective outcome measures to control internal validity. These types of questions are common for clinicians to ask, and thus, the bedside scientist will run across this design frequently, both in literature searches and focused projects.

What were the questions studied in this bedside science project?
Is it safe to use moderate hypothermia in pediatric severe head injury patients? In severe head injured children, are physiologic outcomes better in children treated with a mild hypothermia protocol during their first 3 days of treatment than those treated at normal temperature?

(continues)

Concepts in Action *(continued)*

Why was this research question important?

Injury is the primary cause of death in most pediatric age groups, and severe head injury is a frequent cause. The lifetime disability that may result can be devastating, and death is not uncommon. Because of this, there is a strong research focus on anything that can contribute to preservation of brain tissue and function in the early stages of treating severe head injury in children.

This question was also important because there had been several, promising adult studies of hypothermia and mild hypothermia used in the treatment of severe head injury.

Who was involved on the research team?

This was a multidisciplinary project team that was led by a pediatric intensivist fellow at an academic medical center in Texas. The primary research team included a senior pediatric intensivist, two neurologists, and a pediatric intensive care unit nurse. The team leader also engaged the support of his physician colleagues, advanced practice nurses, respiratory therapists, and pediatric intensive care unit staff nurses.

What were the methods that were planned?

Subjects considered for enrollment in this project were children less than 18 years of age who were admitted to the Pediatric Intensive Care Unit at a children's medical center in Texas over a 13-month period. Children were eligible who were treated for a severe closed traumatic brain injury that occurred up to 6 hours earlier. Subjects were enrolled if they had an admission Glasgow Coma Scale score of 8 or less and underwent insertion of an intracranial pressure (ICP) monitor because they met established criteria for ICP monitoring. Exclusion criteria included clinical brain death, cardiopulmonary arrest before admission, existing ventricular shunts, markedly unstable hemodynamic status, or any condition in which there is an unusual susceptibility or predisposition to bleeding.

The study participants were evaluated in the pediatric intensive care unit for a maximum of 5 days or until ICP monitoring was discontinued, death occurred, or support was withdrawn. Informed consent was obtained from a parent or guardian before enrollment. This study was approved by a university-based institutional review board.

Concepts in Action *(continued)*

Study Protocol

All study patients had ICP monitoring catheters placed on arrival in the pediatric intensive care unit to measure ICP continuously. Using an indwelling arterial catheter, arterial blood pressure was continuously measured.

Group Assignment

After enrollment, the children were randomized to either the normothermia or hypothermia group using a "randomization of pairs" method. In this type of randomization, the first subject is randomly assigned, and the second subject assignment is always the opposite of the first group. For example, if a patient is randomly assigned to the moderate hypothermia group, then the next patient will automatically be assigned the normal temperature group. This assures that the assumptions of randomization are met while still assuring that both groups get an equal number of patients.

Intervention Protocol

All children in the study were placed on a cooling blanket, and their temperature was measured with a rectal temperature probe. For the normothermia treatment group, rectal temperatures were maintained between 36.5°C and 37.5°C during the entire study period. Antipyretics were given if they were indicated. Children in the hypothermia group were kept at 32°C to 34°C, after being lowered to that level over a 4-hour period after admission. This was then maintained for 48 hours, and then patients were warmed to normal temperature over a 12-hour period, at not greater than 1°C every hour for 12 hours.

Intracranial Pressure Management

All patients received usual and supplemental drugs used to manage intracranial pressure during the first 48 hours after their injury. This included continuous infusions of sedatives, analgesics, and neuromuscular blocking agents. They were continued after that period if needed but were usually discontinued after the patient was extubated. The head was positioned in a neutral position, with a 30-degree elevation of the head of the bed. Adequate intravascular volumes, oxygen saturation, and blood pressure were carefully maintained using standard treatment protocols for children in both experimental groups.

(continues)

Concepts in Action *(continued)*

Cerebral physiology was monitored using a standard-sized (4-French) jugular venous bulb catheter inserted in the right subclavian vein, with the tip in the right internal jugular venous bulb. While designing this project—and knowing that there were no established ICP treatment thresholds for children—the study team chose to use conventional treatment thresholds that were already defined for adults.

Physiological and Functional Outcome Measures

Measurements of ICP and cerebral perfusion pressure were taken and stored every minute, giving an astounding 1,400 measurements per patient per day. This gave the researchers a large sample size of measures for analysis. Arterial and jugular venous blood gases, electrolytes (sodium, potassium, chloride, and bicarbonate), ionized calcium, and lactate were monitored every 4 hours as additional measures of cerebral physiology. The arterial jugular venous oxygen content difference and lactate oxygen index were calculated every 4 hours from the blood gas data. Because blood gas values depend on temperature, all blood gas values were corrected for patient temperature. A scoring system was used to rate the various forms of therapy used to control ICP (therapeutic intensity score). For example, supplemental sedation and analgesia received 1 point for each dose administered, and supplemental neuromuscular blockade received 2 points for each dose. Brief hyperventilation episodes scored 1 point. Administration of mannitol scored 3 points, and barbiturates scored 10 points. Values were totaled every 24 hours during the study period.

To evaluate the safety of the hypothermic intervention, the team measured white blood cell count, hemoglobin concentration, hematocrit, platelet count, prothrombin time, partial thromboplastin time, and fibrinogen daily. On a daily basis, they also evaluated measures of liver function, pancreatic function, and renal function tests.

At 3, 6, and 12 months after injury, cognitive and functional outcomes were assessed using three commonly used scores: (1) Glasgow Outcome Score, (2) Pediatric Overall Performance Category, and (3) Pediatric Cerebral Performance Category scales. A clinical nurse research coordinator, who was blinded to the patient's treatment group, performed the evaluation and scoring.

Concepts in Action *(continued)*

Results

This study answered the primary research question when moderate hypothermia is maintained within 6 hours of acute traumatic brain injury trauma in children and then maintained for at least 48 hours, there is a significant decrease in the severity of intracranial hypertension. The second question (is it safe?) was also answered, showing that mild hypothermia treatment was not associated with any more adverse events than in the normal temperature group.

What were the challenges that were faced?

This project was challenging to complete because it was tough to integrate this project within the trauma system—that is, convincing the trauma surgeons to allow these patients to be enrolled in the study. It was also challenging to complete enrollment within the 6-hour time constraint, as many of the patients had to be transferred from a distance and often other serious associated injuries needed to be addressed in addition to the head injury.

Other challenges included making sure that the staff taking care of the patients was carefully following the study protocol and getting information from a posthospital follow-up.

How was this study used?

As a result of this study, a modified protocol was regularly used in the management of severe head-injured children at both the hospital where this study was done and the hospital where the pediatric intensive care unit intensivist later worked. It is currently under consideration for inclusion in the updated pediatric severe head injury guideline undergoing development by a panel of experts.

How was it communicated internally and to larger audiences?

This study was shared internally at a monthly pediatric intensive care unit research lecture with a multidisciplinary group of physicians, nurses, respiratory therapists, and pharmacists. It was also shared as a podium presentation at a professional critical care medicine conference and was published in a well-respected and widely read peer-reviewed journal.

Checklist for Evaluating the Research Question

_____ The purpose of the study is explicitly stated.

_____ The introduction provides support for the importance of the study.

_____ The research problem has significance for your clinical practice.

_____ The research question is appropriately refined, focusing on only one concept in each question.

_____ Hypotheses are written appropriately for each inferential statistical test.

_____ The research question includes sufficient detail to identify *who* is the population, *what* will be measured, *how* will it be measured, and *when* will it be measured.

CHAPTER 4

Scan the Literature

In this chapter, you will learn to
• Search for an available practice guideline • Participate knowledgeably in a systematic review process • Develop a search strategy and conduct a literature search • Construct a literature search for a bedside science project • Strengthen your literature reviews

*"Oh, I will just do a quick literature search." With access to elec-tronic sources for literature, this seems reasonable. After all, the topic—preventing staff's injuries that are caused by lifting—must have a lot of research written about it. You want to build a case for eliminating the lifting that injures so many clinicians, and thus, you need some evidence to back your proposal. While reading through a list of abstracts and the few available full-text articles, however, you are disappointed. Although all of the articles are current and somewhat related to the topic, none gives you the necessary infor-mation. Information on safety is available, but not on injury preven-tion, as you had hoped. Thus, you use more specific key words such as **health care**, **injury**, and **prevention** but are still not get-ting what you want. This is getting frustrating and time consuming. The majority of articles focus on the prevention of patient injuries, and very little is available on staff injury.*

You have a colleague in safety, so you give him a call. You hit pay dirt! He tells you about some extensive Veterans Administra-

tion (VA) studies on staff injuries related to moving patients. He calls the issues "Safe Patient Movement" and shows you the VA Web site that lists multiple studies. Several systematic reviews are published in peer-reviewed journals. The reference lists from the articles are a gold mine of related articles. While looking at the citations, you notice that much of the earlier work was done in the manufacturing and airline industries. You had only considered health care journals; you tuck a thought in the back of your mind not to be so narrow in your search focus in the future.

You realize your poorly focused question may have contributed to the low return of articles. After reading some of the articles, you refine your question to read, "In hospital employees, what staff activities are associated with the highest injury rates?" Armed with your specific question and the new information from the VA articles, you find 36 relevant articles using electronic databases. You find some good operational definitions and a couple of good measurement instruments. One of them even has a design that you think you could replicate in your facility.

Many people think of the literature search as a necessary evil. It takes time to find articles and read abstracts. It takes more time, and sometimes money, to obtain the full-text articles of the most promising abstracts. You can erroneously report that "a dearth of literature on the topic" exists if you are not meticulous and creative in how you approach your literature search. Because of the tremendous number of published studies available (roughly 2 million articles are published every year), each idea is best approached as though evidence already exists. Searching the literature requires you to be part scientist and part detective. Much like a detective uses evidence, the literature is the scientist's way to build a case. Similar to the way evidence is evaluated for relevance in the courtroom, scientists use standards to rate the literature. In a court of law, circumstantial evidence is not as strong as direct evidence because we cannot weigh the effects of random events. Similarly, descriptive studies are not as strong as randomized control trials because we cannot consider the effects of error. Just as evidence can be used in the courtroom to dramatically change a defendant's life, so it is in the science world. Evidence can prevent death and save a life. Its evaluation should not be taken lightly.

Searching the literature is an important part of the research process, and yet it is often considered just a task to be done so that you can get on to the "real" work of research. Think of the evidence as previous experience. If you have a patient with a complicated problem or a serious prognosis, start by reviewing their history and comparing their case to others in your experience. Similarly, you would not begin a research project without knowledge of what has already been found. A systematic and careful search of the literature is crucial in helping you define the question, choose the best possible design, and apply the answers to your practice.

The prospect of a thorough literature search can be daunting for the bedside scientist. The literature review requires access to electronic databases and hardcopy journals, knowledge of search terms, and a critical evaluation of research studies. The search may result in what appears to be an unmanageable quantity of articles to read. The researcher may be tempted to conduct a cursory search, focusing on articles that can be retrieved full text from electronic sources. Although it is a time-consuming process, a thorough literature review can eventually save you time by giving you ideas to focus your question, design your study, and formulate the details of your research. You may even find that a practice guideline already exists, helping you implement a practice change without the need to conduct the research yourself.

DETERMINE WHETHER A GUIDELINE EXISTS

Over the past decade, evidence-based guidelines have become an important source of best practices. A practice guideline uses research findings as a basis for clinician decisions about diagnosis, action, and interaction with patients. Most guidelines are multidisciplinary in nature to reflect the team who will use the guideline. The best place to begin searching for guidelines is the National Guideline Clearinghouse at www.guidelines.gov. Other good sources are professional organizations and peer-reviewed journals, which can be found using database search engines such as OVID, CINAHL, MEDLINE, and Cochrane Reviews.

If a guideline does exist, you will still need to review it carefully. Ask yourself these questions:

- Does this guideline fit my patient population?
- Is this guideline compatible with my setting and level of care?
- Do we have the resources to implement and follow this guideline?
- Are all aspects of this guideline supported by a high level of evidence?
- How will I evaluate compliance with this guideline?
- How will I evaluate the impact of using this guideline on patient outcomes?

If a guideline does not exist for your clinical care question, consider developing your own. This is best accomplished with a multidisciplinary team of clinicians who commonly care for these patients.

RESOURCES FOR GUIDELINE DEVELOPMENT

Some excellent resources that are free to the public are available for guideline development. The Web site (www.guidelines.gov) has numerous links to resources for guideline development and synthesis. One of the best ways to learn how to develop a guideline is to review the elements of a good one that already exists. It will demonstrate the steps that you need to take to develop your own. Most guidelines are organized in a fairly standard way for ease of reading, understanding, and use. Some standard elements that you can expect to see in most guidelines are as follows:

- *Scope statement:* The scope statement provides a review of the background of the problem and the purpose of the guideline. The scope statement can help you to determine whether the guideline will reasonably apply to your setting.
- *The research question:* The research question should be clearly stated, including the population to be studied and the problem that is addressed. Practice guidelines are most commonly focused on prevention, treatment, screening, or diagnosis of clinical problems.
- *The rating method:* The standards used for rating the evidence for methodological quality should be explicit. Table 4-1 presents a common evidence rating scheme.
- *The search strategy:* Elements of the search strategy that are generally reported include the keywords used for the search and the ways the search was conducted (e.g., electronic databases, hand searches, or review of reference lists).
- *The guideline development team:* The members of the guideline development team, their affiliations, and their credentials should be reported. Any sponsors that may reflect potential conflicts of interest should be described.
- *The recommendations:* The bulk of the guideline should focus here. The recommendations will generally include applications to clinical practice as well as an individual rating for each recommendation. If a recommendation applies only to a subgroup, that should be reported here.
- *Identifying information and availability:* The source of the guideline and how copies are requested are described in the guideline.

It is ideal to find an existing practice guideline so that you can implement changes in clinical practice quickly and with confidence in their scientific basis. It is not always possible, however, to find a guideline that fits your patients and setting or to find a guideline at all. In this case, you may need to conduct a systematic review to develop your own guideline or to form the

Table 4-1   A Common Evidence Rating Scheme

Rating	The Evidence
I: Highest Quality	Evidence obtained from at least one properly designed randomized, controlled trial or a systematic review or a meta-analysis of randomized, controlled trials
IIa:	Evidence obtained from well-designed controlled trials without randomization
IIb:	Evidence obtained from well-designed cohort or case-control analytic studies, preferably from more than one center or research group
IIc:	Evidence from multiple time series with or without the intervention (Dramatic results in uncontrolled experiments [such as the results of the introduction of penicillin treatment in the 1940s] could also be regarded as this type of evidence.)
III:	Evidence obtained from a systematic review of case-control studies
IV:	Evidence based on opinions of respected authorities based on clinical experience, descriptive studies (survey or qualitative designs), case studies, or reports of expert committees
V:	Evidence obtained from an expert's biased opinion that is not supported by published research studies or is based on assumptions about how a patient is likely to respond physiologically

From the Mouths of Bedside Scientists: How Is Literature Used in Research Design?

What are some things you have learned from your literature search that helped with your study design?

I always look at the way others have studied what I am trying to study and at their limitations. I have probably used information in the limitation section more than anything else to avoid problems with my study design. One example that comes to mind is a study that ended with very low follow-up numbers because they were trying to do the follow-up in a student population when most of the students were home on summer break. You have to pay attention to the smaller details, and sometimes you will not think of these on your own.

I learned that reading full-text articles instead of just abstracts is necessary. You can only tell so much from an abstract. The full-text article gives you the lowdown on every aspect of the study. A few times I have been very surprised that the great outcome reported in an abstract does not look so great once you read the methods of that study.

How have you used literature to develop a guideline, protocol, or policy and procedure?

Our unit is in the middle of updating all of our policies and procedures (which is a pain), and it has been very enlightening to find that many things in our old procedures are not based on evidence of any sort. Although frustrating, it has also been a great lesson. We have actually changed several policies and thrown some in the trash after we reviewed and critically appraised the literature.

Writing a protocol is painful because of the time and searching challenges that are involved. Then you have to figure out ways to help all of the members of an interdisciplinary clinical team be compliant and actually *use* the protocol. After you do the work, however, the results can be pretty amazing. I think a side effect of a good protocol is better staff and patient satisfaction (which may be my next study). I just know it takes so much of the guesswork out of care, especially when you have a large team.

basis for a focused research project. Keep in mind that a systematic review of the literature is not for the faint of heart; it is for the clinician who is willing to be a detective and put in the time to find, make sense of, and apply the literature.

A SCIENTIFIC BASIS FOR PRACTICE: THE SYSTEMATIC REVIEW

Systematic reviews are important to bedside scientists as a way of synthesizing current research literature to support informed decisions. A systematic review is a process of determining the best possible evidence for a clinical practice by identifying, appraising, and synthesizing the relevant literature. Medical information on many topics may be extensive but of dubious quality. Readily available research may include a number of peer-reviewed journal articles or papers from an electronic database, but the selection of studies may not be representative of the best literature available and may not tell the entire story. A systematic review accomplishes a structured and extremely thorough search of the research literature for a specific topic, using a strategy that ensures retrieval of all relevant studies.

Authors of systematic reviews refine the search and select only those papers that measure up to established quality standards for inclusion in final recommendations. A systematic review process provides a step-by-step procedure for summarizing the otherwise unmanageable quantities of research available for guiding clinical practice.

Words such as *thorough, orderly, organized, efficient, logical,* and *methodical* describe how you need to think about the systematic review process. Every systematic review requires careful search methods, research appraisal skills, and clinical expertise of those working on the review team. The actual literature search is a critical aspect of the systematic review. If the search process is done incorrectly, the results could possibly be biased or could provide an incomplete evidence base for the review.

The literature search for a systematic review is constructed to maximize the relevant literature retrieved and to deal effectively with potentially biasing factors. Clinicians are well advised to consult with a medical librarian for help in developing literature search skills. Expert searchers are an important part of the team and are, in fact, crucial throughout the systematic review process—from the development of the proposal and research question to publication of recommendations.

Develop the Research Question

When working with a systematic review team, the first step is to evaluate the question to determine whether a systematic review is indicated. Systematic reviews are appropriate for clinical practices if
- There is a disparity between the current clinical practice and the scientific literature.
- The benefits of current treatments are uncertain.

- The cost-effectiveness of current practice has not been demonstrated.
- Current practice is based on evidence that is primarily anecdotal.
- Variations in current practice are common.

If a systematic review is indicated, begin by developing a specific research question. The research question should specify the population of interest, the focus of the review (prevention, therapy, screening, or diagnosis), and the outcomes of interest. All of these elements will be used in formulating the search strategy.

Define Specific Search Criteria

Develop specific search criteria to identify the literature that will be used for the review. The aim is to generate as comprehensive a list as possible of primary studies, both published and unpublished, that may be suitable for answering the question. Inclusion and exclusion criteria are developed to identify those articles that will help answer the question. These criteria generally include the population, the interventions, the outcomes, and the study types. Making these decisions *a priori* (before the study begins) helps keep the search free of bias.

Refine the criteria to maximize the relevance of the literature that is retrieved. These refinements may include characteristics such as age groups, gender, or time periods for the search. Develop a list of key words that will be used for the search. Consider each element in the research question in determining the key word list and then broaden the key word list by identifying synonyms and variants for each word. For example, a synonym for *neonate* might be *newborn*, and a variant is *neonatal*. If, at any point in the review process, any criteria are changed, keep all of your team members aware of these changes, as they may influence the search strategy and search results. The list of key words will form the basis for a consistent approach to the search of the literature, regardless of the source.

Select Key Search Resources

Select the key sources for the search based on accessibility, resources, and your team's search skill. Use all of the electronic databases available to you, as well as Web sites, including those of professional organizations. Common healthcare databases are OVID, CINAHL (the Cumulative Index to Nursing and Allied Health Literature), MEDLINE, PubMED, PEDro (physiotherapy), and PsychINFO. Do not ignore resources that contain the "gray literature" or abstracts from conferences and dissertations. Although studies in these databases are not published in journals, they are still peer reviewed and can be particu-

Hitting the Stacks

Pengel, Maher, and Refshauge (2002) conducted a systematic review of conservative interventions for subacute low back pain. They identified studies through searches of 18 databases, and thus, they needed a clear plan for focusing on those studies with the most relevance for their clinical question. The authors used five inclusion criteria to narrow the field:

> 1) *Design* Only randomized controlled trials were included. 2) *Study population* Subjects with subacute non-specific low back pain with or without referral to the leg. . . . 3) *Interventions* All types of conservative treatment were included (i.e. surgery was excluded). 4) *Outcomes* Studies were required to report at least one of the following outcome measures: pain, disability, or return to work. 5) *Language* The study was published in English or Dutch.

Cartwright-Hatton et al. (2004) demonstrated the extensiveness of a systematic review search process in their review of the efficacy of cognitive behavior therapies for childhood anxiety disorders.

> The search for trials comprised [eight] electronic databases; reference lists of reviews and book chapters; and hand search of journals. . . . The reference lists of recent reviews and trials were examined. . . . Journals were selected for hand search as follows: every journal that had published a trial identified by the previous stages [and] journals that were known to publish trials on the treatment of anxiety disorders . . . the content lists of these [13] journals, from January 1990 to August 2003, were hand searched by a child psychiatrist and a trained clinical psychologist using the search terms produced for the electronic search.

Pengel, H., C. Maher, and K. Refshauge. 2002. Systematic review of conservative interventions for subacute low back pain. *Pain Reviews* 9: 153–63.

Cartwright-Hatton, S., C. Roberts, P. Chitsabesan, C. Fothergill, and R. Harrington. 2004. Systematic review of the efficacy of cognitive behaviour therapies for childhood and adolescent anxiety disorders. *British Journal of Clinical Psychology* 43: 421–36.

larly timely. Considering that the average research study takes 3 years from inception to publication, conference proceedings and dissertation abstracts may contain the most up-to-date information about clinical effectiveness.

Decisions about specific resources should be based on a careful evaluation of the relevance of each source to the research question. This is where a medical librarian can be particularly helpful. As you gain experience in this skill, you will be able to identify major studies as well as the leading journals and conferences for your searches. Supplemental techniques can be used to assure that the search is as comprehensive as possible. Examples are hand searching the tables of contents of journals that are directly relevant and "mining" the reference lists of key articles; both are common (although time-intensive) search strategies.

Strive for as comprehensive a search as possible. Do not rely on a single electronic database for a search, as every search can be expected to have less than perfect literature retrieval. Avoid focusing on only those databases that provide full text of articles, as the result may be superficial and incomplete. Relying solely on published articles may introduce bias into the review. The tendency for positive findings to be preferentially published means that the

Another Way to Look at It

The literature review is a common way for a bedside scientist to find the inconsistencies in a clinical process and to plan a study to solve a problem. The review may expose gaps in the current knowledge or may reveal contradictory findings. A study can then be designed that will fill in the gaps and determine conclusively whether a given intervention is effective. Although the literature search can seem daunting, it does not have to be. Approach it as if you are trying to use your experience and the experiences of others to solve a problem.

When I was young, Sunday afternoon dinners at my grandmother's farm were extra special when she made homemade doughnuts. These were not the kind of doughnuts you get at the coffee shop, but rather steaming, rich, melt-in-your mouth pastries. As I got older and my grandmother grew frail, I decided not to lose this family tradition. I asked her for the recipe, and although she gave it to me willingly, mine did not turn out like hers. Part of the problem was precision—her measures were not what I would call standard: "a handful of shortening, then some salt and enough flour to make it hold together." I kept the recipe but figured that the doughnuts were a thing of the past when my grandmother passed away.

A couple of years ago, while at a family dinner with my cousins, I made the comment that I would surely love one of grandma's doughnuts. I discovered that I was not the only one of my generation to get the recipe from her; indeed, several of us had versions of it written down and tucked in our recipe boxes. We decided to bring them to the next dinner,

published literature is biased. Relying only on studies in print gives an exaggerated impression of how well a treatment works because studies that found no effect are less likely to be published. As you do your search, you will be responsible for guarding against bias in the search. A database-only search would generally be considered a mark of low quality.

A comprehensive selection of sources for a systematic review often includes two or more bibliographic databases such as MEDLINE and CINAHL, a trials registry, conference proceedings, specialized subject bibliographies, reference lists of review articles, and contact with experts in the field. Expect some redundancy as you make your way to a comprehensive list of citations relevant to your question.

Another Way to Look at It *(continued)*

compare notes, and see whether we could come up with the definitive directions.

We had six different versions of the recipe. No two of them were the same. One recipe had salt in it; another had no salt but a lot of baking powder. One used butter instead of shortening. Three called for kneading before rolling out the dough, but two specifically said to pat the dough flat without kneading. The temperatures listed for the cooking oil were all different. As we compared the recipes side by side, however, some commonalities were apparent—some ingredients were in all of them in relatively the same amounts. The comparison also revealed some gaps and inconsistencies, but these were pretty easy to find when we had all of the recipes in front of us.

We decided that we would take the most consistent set of ingredients and start experimenting with the various aspects of the recipe that were unclear. After about four attempts—and a whole lot of taste testing by the kids—we finally hit on the flavor and texture we remembered. We now have the definitive "Grandma's Doughnuts" recipe in a form that *can* be passed on to our kids and on to theirs.

The literature search can serve your research equally well. The literature will not likely answer your question, but it will give you an idea of what has already been found and what results seem to recur. It may also reveal the gaps and inconsistencies that need further study. The search can help you to focus your study on these gaps until the whole story emerges.

Using Databases Effectively

A comprehensive search requires an understanding of databases and how they work. It is vital for the searcher to understand the differences between fields. For example, the subject heading (sh) field and the publication type (pt) field contain very different information. An article with the subject heading of randomized controlled trial is an article *about* randomized controlled trials, whereas an article with the publication type of randomized controlled trial is an *actual* randomized controlled trial. An awareness of the meaning and implications of searching different fields will help determine the quality of your search strategy.

Various limiters and tags are available on most major databases. For example, a search can be limited to a publication type, a particular age group, a span of years, or a single language. Limiters can help focus a search and reduce the number of irrelevant citations but may also result in an incomplete citation list. For these reasons, it is always helpful to have a medical librarian actually serve on the systematic review team.

The Retrieval Process: The First Screening

The objective of the search is to retrieve as much relevant material as possible. Most of the studies will be retrieved from electronic databases. Just as a researcher can identify weaknesses in a study design through a pilot study, the systematic reviewer can identify problems with a search strategy through a first search. Conduct a trial search on one of the major health care databases (e.g., CINAHL or MEDLINE) and generate an initial list of citations. This list will include many articles that are not relevant or that do not meet the inclusion criteria. On the other hand, it may be missing key articles. A good way to evaluate the retrieved set is to verify that major studies identified by the subject experts appear on the list. The team can use the results of this first search to refine the search criteria before proceeding to the full search. After the reviewers are satisfied with the search strategy, it can be customized and executed in the indexing language of the other databases to be searched.

The results of the database searches are usually quite large compared with the results from a focused clinical query. An early challenge is to make sense of a large list of citations. Figure 4-1 illustrates the process of narrowing the search results until only the best relevant articles remain. Software is available to manage the citations (e.g., Reference Manager or EndNote), which convert references from different sources to a common format and removes duplicates.

Keep careful counts at each step of the screening process. These citation counts are important for final reporting, when all identified citations must be

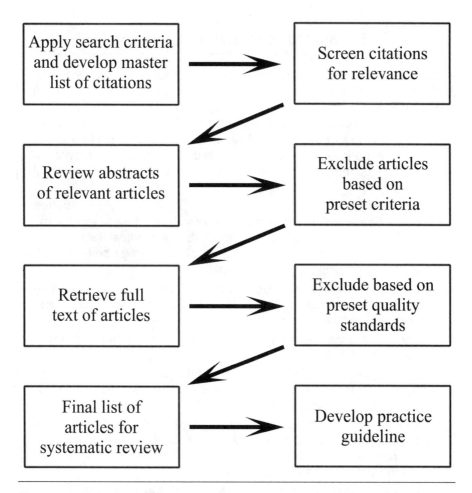

Figure 4-1   A process for focusing the literature for a systematic review.

accounted for (i.e., whether they were duplicates, screened out by reviewers, or ultimately included in the review). Documenting the reasons that articles were included or excluded helps maintain the internal validity of the review and minimizes bias.

The various stages of the review may take from several hours to several days to complete. The initial list will be pared down when articles that are obviously irrelevant or do not meet inclusion criteria are removed. More articles will be excluded after a review of the research abstracts. The final list for the review will be substantially shorter than the first list; thus, do not be daunted by the initial number of citations to review. It is easy to get discouraged by the

Strengthen Your Literature Searches

It is easy to see the literature search as a task that has to be done in order to get at the "real" work of research. If it is done well, however, a thorough review of previous work can actually save time in the long run. The literature search can help you to focus your research question, develop the details of your study design, and put your study in a larger context. Doing a literature search requires time and a bit of frustration tolerance—but these hints can help you get the most from this critical step.

• Early in the process, involve a medical librarian in your literature search. Searching the literature is a methodical science, and the expertise a librarian brings can be invaluable. A medical librarian can help you find databases and develop a search strategy, both of which can improve your chances of success.

• Go from general to specific in your search strategy. Look for studies on your overall topic first, and then search for research that is more specific to your unique question.

• If you find a key study that is similar to your question, "mine" its reference list.

• Resist the urge to look only at full-text databases. You will miss valuable studies and wind up with an incomplete literature review if you focus on easily accessible articles.

• Use a broad range of sources, including "gray literature," such as conference proceedings and dissertation abstracts. Do not ignore hand searches of the most relevant journals, as you may find articles that were missed in your electronic sources.

• Rely on primary sources—in other words, the original studies—instead of quotes or summaries from other articles. Studies may be misquoted and findings reported incorrectly, and thus, you have to go to the source to be sure that you have the findings right.

amount of time and effort the searching will take, but the work is worth it. Every aspect of the search is of value as you develop and refine your study.

The Final Review: A Focus on Methodologic Quality

After all of the citations and abstracts have been reviewed for relevance to the research question, full-text articles are retrieved of the final studies on the list. Each study will be appraised for methodologic quality and given an "evidence rating." Standards for methodological soundness are set before the actual review begins to prevent researcher bias. The team then applies the standards to the articles on the final list and the evidence from each is rated and summarized into one large document. The most common elements of methodologic quality to evaluate are as follows:

- Sampling strategy: Is the sample representative? Was there less than 20% attrition? Was the sample selected or assigned to groups randomly?
- Measurement: Were the measurement instruments valid, reliable, and consistently applied?
- Internal validity: Were alternative explanations for the results controlled, eliminated, or accounted for in some way?
- Statistical conclusions: Was statistical significance achieved with the data? Was the effect size large enough to be clinically meaningful?
- External validity: Were conclusions drawn appropriately about generalizing the study to other populations?

The final summary of evidence from articles with acceptable methodologic quality is the systematic review. A review is a tremendous amount of work and will only make a contribution to the body of clinical knowledge if it is communicated to a wider audience. Publication in a peer-reviewed journal, evaluation by an expert systematic review team, or submission to the National Guideline Clearinghouse is the final step for a review. Your team's findings can then be used by other busy clinicians to guide or change practice and improve patient care.

THE LITERATURE REVIEW FOR A BEDSIDE SCIENTIST PROJECT

For some bedside science projects, no practice guideline may be available, and a systematic review may not be indicated. Ideally, you will find a literature review on your topic or a similar topic. If not, then you can begin your own careful search of the literature. Although the literature review for a focused research process does not require the depth that is typical of a systematic review, it does require a methodical approach. For a bedside science project, rather than using the literature to make recommendations for clinical practice, you are using prior research to build a case for the importance of your study. The literature also serves to help focus your research question and plan the study design. You may even be lucky enough to find a study that you can replicate, saving you the work of planning and designing every element of a research project.

Even though the literature review for a bedside science project is not as involved as a systematic review, several review steps can help you find good support for your study. Use your research question to identify key search terms and develop a search strategy. Keep track of your search terms and the sources you searched. A good rule of thumb for your minisystematic review is to start with a general review of your overall subject and then move on to specific areas that are unique to your project. For example, a bedside scientist might want to evaluate patient satisfaction and comfort with two pneumatic compression devices used on a trauma unit to decrease deep vein thrombosis (DVT). The general literature review could evaluate all methods used to reduce DVT and then specifically focus on the effectiveness of these two devices. Literature could be retrieved that reports the prevalence of DVT in trauma patients and the risks to the patient if one occurs. Information about the cost of a DVT and the cost-effectiveness of the devices could also be studied. The researcher could search related literature on what contributes to patient comfort and satisfaction. Searches might also be conducted on patient satisfaction with therapeutic devices in general. All of this information, taken together, provides a basis for the importance of the study and guidance for design of the specific research project.

Evaluate Study Credibility

The literature review for a bedside science project is no less rigorous in its standards for study quality than the systematic review. The guidelines for evaluating the credibility of a study, described earlier in this chapter, are applied to a bedside science literature review as well. Although the results are used differently—instead of changing practice, you are providing background and support for your research—the studies you include in your review should be credible. By appraising the validity of studies you review, you will be able to consider whether the research you review relates to your situation.

Writing the Literature Review for a Bedside Science Project

The literature review is a written summary that synthesizes the existing knowledge about a research problem. The task for the bedside scientist is to present and evaluate existing research to provide an overview of the existing knowledge about the topic under study. The literature review should begin with an introduction that places the problem in context by reporting the prevalence and impact of the problem. Background research on your topic is provided next, as is a theoretical basis for your study. Describe studies that are directly and indirectly related to your research question. Be as objective as possible, and present both the strengths and weaknesses of the studies that are reviewed. Studies that are contradictory or that do not support your hypothesis should not be ignored but reported objectively. One of the purposes of bedside science is to clarify previous contradictions, and thus, part of build-

For more depth and detail, try these resources:

Ansani, N.T., G.A. Fedutes-Henderson, S.J. Skledar, R. Branch, C. Sirio, T. Smitherman, and R.J. Weber. 2005. Practical approach to grading evidence for formulary recommendations. *American Journal of Health-System Pharmacy* 62: 1498–52.

Atkins, D., K. Fink, and J. Slutsky. 2005. Better information for better health care: The Evidence-Based Practice Center program and the Agency for Healthcare Research and Quality. *Annals of Internal Medicine* 142(12 Pt. 2): 1035–41.

Drake, R.E., E.A. Latimer, H.S. Leff, G.J. McHugo, and B.J. Burns. 2004. What is evidence? *Child and Adolescent Psychiatric Clinics of North America* 13: 717–28.

Glasziou, P., L. Irwiq, C. Bain, and G. Colditz. 2005. *Systematic Reviews in Health Care: A Practical Guide.* London: Cambridge University Press.

Khan, K.S., R. Kunz, J. Kleijnen, and G. Antes. 2003. *Systematic Reviews to Support Evidence-Based Medicine: How to Review and Apply Findings of Healthcare Research.* London: Royal Society of Medicine Press.

Locke, L. F., S.J. Silverman, and W.W. Spirduso. 2004. *Reading and Understanding Research.* Thousand Oaks, CA: Sage Publications.

Melnyk, B., and E. Fineout-Overholt. 2004. *Evidence-Based Practice in Nursing and Healthcare: A Guide to Best Practice.* Philadelphia: Lippincott, Williams & Wilkins.

Santaguida, P.L., M. Helfand, and P. Raina. 2005. Challenges in systematic reviews that evaluate drug efficacy or effectiveness. *Annals of Internal Medicine* 142(12 Pt. 2): 1066–72.

Shekelle, P.G., S.C. Morton, M.J. Suttorp, N. Buscemi, and C. Friesen. 2005. Challenges in systematic reviews of complementary and alternative medicine topics. *Annals of Internal Medicine* 142(12 Pt. 2): 1042–7.

Swan, B.A., and R.F. Boruch. 2004. Quality of evidence: usefulness in measuring the quality of health care. *Medical Care* 42(2 Suppl): 12–20.

Wong, S.S., N.L. Wilczynski, and R.B. Haynes. 2004. Developing optimal search strategies for detecting clinically relevant qualitative studies in MEDLINE. *Medinfo* 11: 311–6.

ing the case is revealing the inconsistencies and gaps in the current knowledge about your question.

The purpose of the literature review is to build a case for the importance of your research, and thus, a logical argument should unfold that leads the reader to understand why your study needs to be done. Very few opinions from the literature should be presented, and the researcher's opinion should be virtually undetectable. If a researcher's bias is obvious in the literature review, then the reader will have little confidence in the ability of the researcher to remain objective during the study.

The literature review does not need to be extensive but should present the most relevant information about your topic. It is not necessary to review every study ever done but rather the studies that have the most significance for your project. The literature review should conclude with a summary of the most current knowledge about your topic, leading to a logical conclusion that your study is important and relevant for clinical practice.

SUMMARY

Scanning the literature is a critical part of the research process that takes skill, a thoughtful plan, and careful execution. Inconsistencies in current practice are common subjects for literature review. The first effort should be to find an existing practice guideline. If none exists, then a systematic review may be appropriate. Specific steps are required for a systematic review, including developing a research question, defining search criteria, selecting and using key search resources, screening initial citations, and appraising a final list of studies for methodologic quality. The outcome of a systematic review is a summary of the best available evidence for a clinical practice. A bedside science project also requires a review of the literature, although it is not generally as in-depth as a systematic review. A critique of the literature obtained from searches results in a better knowledge and understanding of issues related to your topic and helps you to design the best possible study.

Concepts in Action

Implementing an evidence-based protocol to guide practice does not just happen. It takes careful thought and planning and often impacts more than one clinical discipline. In the following example, the protocol implementation process began with a felt and demonstrated need and the desire to make the process "better." Although there was little formal literature on the topic, the team used the available evidence and consulted similar providers to draw conclusions about effective diagnoses, treatments, and admission decisions. The team eventually answered the research question with the development of a protocol and a treatment

Concepts in Action *(continued)*

algorithm. As you read this example, consider key aspects to keep in mind when you develop and implement an evidence-based protocol in your own setting.

What were the questions studied in this bedside science project?
What are the components of a multidisciplinary treatment protocol for mild traumatic brain injury (MTBI) in children ages 9 to 17 years and in adults ages 18 to 65 years for use in a level 1 trauma center emergency department (ED), a trauma neurological intensive care unit (NICU), and a pediatric intensive care unit (PICU) of an east coast academic community hospital?

Why was this research question important?
An MTBI or a "concussion" is a common reason for hospitalization; it is ranked third behind only abrasions and contusions as the most common ICD-9 code resulting in hospital admissions. In the pediatric age group, MTBIs and extremity fractures are *the* most common admission diagnoses. Despite the prevalence of this condition, there was no uniform agreement on effective treatment, the role of diagnostic tests, and when to admit an MTBI patient for inpatient care.

At this hospital, the necessity for a guideline was established on review of data from a trauma database that identified significant variability in treatment of MTBI patients. The multidisciplinary team responsible for care of these patients also reported an anecdotal need for consistent care guidelines for these patients—especially because the care of these patients required resources in trauma units, NICUs, and PICUs.

Who was involved on the research team?
An adult trauma surgeon (chief of trauma surgery) and a trauma nurse coordinator—formerly a PICU nurse—were the drivers of this project and engaged a multidisciplinary team. The team consisted of a trauma surgeon, several neurosurgeons and pediatric intensivists, a pediatric nurse practitioner, a pediatric nurse educator, PICU staff nurses, and the pediatric trauma nurse coordinator.

What were the methods that were planned?
The initial plan was to find an evidence-based guideline and implement it. The team conducted a thorough search of the literature, contacted
(continues)

Concepts in Action *(continued)*

multiple professional organizations, and consulted other level 1 trauma centers, but no protocol was found. The team then decided to create a protocol based on existing evidence.

Finding the Scientific Evidence

Building a protocol from scratch can be tough. This team began by identifying key areas of treatment variability. This focused the team on the treatment that happens in the ED and the responsibilities of each member of the care team and each department. Inconsistencies were identified in admission decisions, and also in the treatments that happen in the trauma unit, the NICU, or the PICU. Team members consulted other level 1 trauma centers and PICUs to determine their usual methods for dealing with these aspects of care.

The key areas identified were as follows:

• Definition, epidemiology, and clinical characteristics of MTBI

• Role of computed tomography and neuropsychiatric testing in the diagnosis and management of MTBI

• Guidelines for hospital admission versus evaluation and discharge to home

• Process for identification and treatment of post-traumatic and emotional symptoms in patients with an MTBI

Members of the team, particularly the PICU nurse trauma coordinator, used these areas as key search terms to find scientific literature related to the care of this population.

What were the challenges that were faced?

This project was challenging because the care of MTBI involved multiple disciplines, several departments, and a heterogeneous population with a wide age range (9 to 65 years). Initially, only 38 useful articles were found on the topic, and only a few of these articles dealt with children. Of these, only 11 were considered scientific research, with only one level I evidence article. Seven were judged to be level II evidence, and three were determined to be level III evidence articles (see Table 4.1). Because so little evidence was available, the team focused on diagnosis, treatment, and criteria for inpatient admission and postponed strategies for addressing emotional issues for a later study.

Concepts in Action *(continued)*

What were the key steps of the protocol, and how was it used?

Using the literature that was available, the information from consultations, and professional experience with MTBI patients, the protocol team defined the following steps:

1. Apply inclusion criteria to determine whether the patient meets the requirements for a diagnosis of MTBI.
2. Administer a screening tool for a cognitive evaluation.
3. Use the appropriate treatment protocol for those who are diagnosed as MTBI.
4. Determine whether the patient meets the criteria for inpatient admission.
5. Apply criteria for safe discharge, including standardized follow-up instructions.

The details of the protocol appear in Table 4-2.

After the protocol was developed, the first step toward implementation was development of a treatment algorithm based on the protocol. A treatment algorithm can facilitate ease of use in practice. This algorithm used a six-step process guided by five "yes or no" questions and one positive versus negative computerized tomography scan screening question. Because all key clinicians involved in the care of patients with MTBI were also involved in the development of the protocol, implementing the protocol went fairly smoothly. It was communicated at both leadership and staff meetings, and a go-live date was set.

The Trauma Database

Data from the protocol algorithm were collected on every MTBI patient and entered into a large trauma outcome database by a trauma data collector. This was an important aspect of protocol implementation and allowed the team to evaluate outcomes of care in this population. After a brief pilot phase for clinicians to familiarize themselves with the protocol algorithm, 100% compliance was eventually reached.

As the protocol became embedded in practice, subsequent reports of treatment compliance and outcomes of MTBI patients were shared with the entire multidisciplinary team on a regular basis and used to guide

(continues)

Table 4-2   Detailed Protocol for Management of MTBI

MTBI inclusion criteria (level II–III evidence)
Blunt mechanism
Brief neurologic deficit, for example, if loss of consciousness (LOC) less than 20 minutes or brief retrograde amnesia (amnestic event)
Glasgow Coma Score (GCS) of 13 to 15
No focal neurologic deficit on exam
No intracranial complications (e.g., seizure, unexplained vomiting for more than 12 hours)
Normal brain computerized tomography, including no skull fracture
Ages 9 to 65 years

Use of a moderate concussion head injury (CHI) protocol (level III evidence)
Head computerized tomography for any change in LOC
If patient meets the criteria for severe CHI (see Management of Severe Head Injury Protocol)

Indications to admit to inpatient care (level I–III evidence)
Nonisolated injuries such as multiple teeth/alveolar ridge fractures, open nasal fractures, sinus fractures, orbit, zygoma, other facial fractures, or major scalp lacerations
Inability to radiographically clear the cervical spine
Mini Mental Status Exam (MMSE) of less than 19 if less than 4 years of education, less than 23 if 5 to 8 years of education, and less than 27 if 9 to 12 years of education

Concepts in Action *(continued)*

both process improvement and research studies. Because these data then feed into a larger trauma registry database, the team can track their outcomes against those of other hospitals.

As new information is published in the literature and other evidence-based guidelines appear, the multidisciplinary team has the opportunity to suggest updates to the protocol. In a sense, it is a living document so that the best possible process of care for treatment of MTBI patients is used.

Table 4-2   Detailed Protocol for Management of MTBI *(continued)*

Consultant recommendation to admit the patient, and/or team leader judgment
Exclude minor injuries such as abrasions, lacerations, and sprains/strains that would otherwise be treated with the patient released

Safe discharge criteria include (level II–III evidence)
GCS score of 15
Low-risk symptoms only (level III evidence)
Asymptomatic, headache, dizziness, scalp hematoma, scalp laceration, scalp contusion, and scalp abrasion
Absence of moderate or high-risk criteria (GCS of less than 13)
No drug or alcohol involvement
Reliable adult able to transport and stay with patient, capable of performing serial neurologic exams
Lives within 30 minutes of trauma center (access to phone/transportation)
Telephone at home

Discharge from the trauma unit
Follow-up instructions include discharge packet, forwarding patient's home phone number to the trauma team leader's office (phone number and extension listed).
Patients with mild symptomatology may be excluded at the discretion of the trauma attending. Severe or multiple symptoms require a physiatrist consult (level II and III evidence).

Concepts in Action *(continued)*

How was it communicated internally and to larger audiences?
The use of the protocol was first communicated internally through both unit leadership and staff meetings. Several abstracts were written and presented at national and international conferences about this hospital's experience using the protocol, including patient outcome data from the trauma database. Subsequent studies are planned, including one to look at ways of evaluating and treating posttraumatic stress disorder and emotional symptoms.

Checklist for Evaluating a Literature Review

_____ The literature review relies primarily on the most recent studies.

_____ All or most of the major studies related to the topic of interest are included.

_____ The review can be linked directly and indirectly to the research question.

_____ The review provides support for the importance of the study.

_____ The review is unbiased and includes findings that are conclusive and those that have inconsistencies.

_____ The author's opinion is virtually undetectable.

_____ The review is organized so that a logical unfolding of ideas is apparent that supports the need for the research.

_____ The review ends with a summary of the most important knowledge on the topic.

CHAPTER 5

Solicit Organizational Commitment

In this chapter, you will learn to

- Prepare an application for consideration by the institutional review board
- Develop an informed consent form
- Design a data collection procedure that complies with HIPAA regulations
- Find organizational resources to help with your study
- Strengthen organizational commitment to the success of your study

---

You are angry—justifiably angry. You and six team members designed a superb trial to evaluate a new concoction for wound healing. A colleague who was doing bench research developed the cream. After the Food and Drug Administration's requirements for human testing were met, a colleague contacted you to see whether you wanted to study its effectiveness. The drug, which looked promising, would be free of charge for your patients during the study period. You had no financial interest but would like to see a better treatment for your patients; thus, you agreed.

Some colleagues were asked to join your team to discuss the study. It took more than 6 months for the team to decide how best to test the effectiveness of the product. The group narrowed the question to focus on the population of postsurgical diabetic patients. The team spent hours searching the literature and then more hours evaluating and pooling the information. You literally wrote a systematic review of the existing evidence on postopera-

tive wound healing in patients with diabetes. The team decided that a randomized, placebo-controlled trial would be the best next step. Your team worked hard and developed a strong design.

The team spent many hours conversing with the institutional review board (IRB) administrator and ethicists. At the IRB meeting, which was very intimidating, you and two team members did a nice job of fielding some tough questions. Several weeks later you received formal IRB approval. The final step was to find staff to help.

That was the cause for your anger. Both the nursing administrator and the medical director looked stunned when you showed them your study protocol and the IRB approval letter—no pat on the back for your hard work. In fact, they both said the same thing: you should have come to them before spending time designing the specifics of the study. The medical director asked how you expected to find time to do the study with your busy surgery schedule. Of course, you had expected the residents to enroll patients and order treatments. Bedside nurses could apply the treatment when they gave medications, although 30 minutes four times a day would add up. The nurse administrator asks whether you involved a bedside nurse on your team. How do you know the process will work? How did you estimate the time needed for application of the study drug and placebo? How much total staff time would the study need? Who would pay for all those hours of nursing time?

As you began to estimate the total time that involves residents and nurses, anger begins simmering—and the anger is at yourself. Looking at the numbers, you know there is no way that a busy medical–surgical nurse could be expected to carry out this protocol, no matter how simple it looks on paper. You thought that the 292 patients dictated by the power analysis was a lot but did not think about how much time it would take to treat all of the patients.

Your medical director walks out with you as you shake your head in dismay. She assures you that you have a well-designed and important study. Anything that holds promise to improve wound healing in high-risk patients with diabetes should be studied. She suggests that you will have success with a small pilot that can be used to estimate the time requirements and serve as a basis for grant funding. She suggests a grant writer who can support your team in the grant process. Later that week, you and your team show the wound treatment process to a group of bedside nurses and discover a quicker and better way to apply the treatment protocol.

Every research project requires attention to much more than the scientific aspects for the study to be done well. Ideally, the legal, ethical, economic, and political issues are considered throughout the study design phase. While thinking about the who, what, when, and where of the study, contemplate who is affected by each step and what it will cost in time and money. What looks great on paper sometimes cannot be done because of time or other budget constraints. Project management principles apply to research projects just as they do to other major organizational projects, and that means being concerned with process as well as outcomes.

Unfortunately, sometimes a researcher is so focused on the science of a project that the nonscience issues are left to chance. As our skin cream researcher discovered, science cannot be done well if organizational questions are not addressed simultaneously. The biggest challenges in accomplishing bedside science projects may not be scientific but humanistic. When *plans* must become *action*, then a much larger group of people must be involved and committed to the research. Successful negotiation of this phase requires consideration of these larger organizational considerations. Address these elements as carefully as the scientific design of the study to enhance your chances of success.

ETHICAL ISSUES AND IRB PROCEDURES

Ethics is a fundamental concern in research involving human subjects, and the IRB provides guidance and oversight to assure that studies are ethical. The purpose of the IRB is to assure that proposed research projects are ethically acceptable; their primary focus is protection of the rights of human subjects. These rights focus on assuring that studies are well designed and reasonably able to achieve a goal, that subjects have adequate information to make a decision about participation, and that subjects are not exposed to undue risk.

An onsite IRB, if available, will be an important resource as you develop your research project. The IRB wades through governmental regulatory changes and shares that information with investigators, explaining how it impacts their projects. The documentation requirements of the IRB help to assure that studies are done in an ethically sound manner and that individual human rights are considered. They monitor adverse events during the study, any planned or unplanned study closures, and review reports of results. Recruiting subjects for the study cannot begin until IRB approval is formally received.

The IRB requires that all primary investigators sign an annual conflict of interest statement to assure that they will not benefit from the results in a financial way. This helps to control researcher bias. All members of the investigative team are required to complete an annual course on human protection. Any investigator can complete the National Institutes of Health (NIH) tutorial by visiting this website: http://cme.cancer.gov/clinicaltrials/learning/humanparticipant-protections.asp.

Certain populations of patients require additional protection, including infants and children who are less than 18 years old, mentally impaired individuals, pregnant women, and persons who are incarcerated. If you submit an application for a study on one of these vulnerable groups, expect additional scrutiny of the informed consent, procedures, and methods that minimize risk.

Full Board Review

The IRB is comprised of clinical and research experts and sometimes key community members (e.g., clergy, judges, business owners, and college professors). Legal consultants are also available to the IRB. The IRB chair is usually a clinician–scientist with extensive clinical and research experience.

The IRB will carefully look at every aspect of a project. Expect particular focus on

- The research design: Is it clear what the investigator is going to do? Is the study design adequate to address the research question? Are necessary controls in place?
- The impact on the patient: Are the risks to the patient outweighed by the benefits to the patient? Is an appropriate informed consent procedure in place?
- The investigator's command of the subject: Does it make sense to do this study in this population of patients? Is there a good understanding of the clinical issues involved?

The IRB application is formalized information about your study; it forces you and your team to carefully consider every aspect of your project. The consent form is your way of assuring that every patient has the chance to understand fully what the study is about and how it impacts him or her (Table 5-1). A copy of a thorough informed consent appears in Appendix A.

Before the IRB meeting, you will have many chances to interact with the IRB office. Take advantage of your interactions. Ask questions, and follow the guidelines that they provide. Seek out an ethicist as a resource. You can get feedback on the wording of your consent and advice to strengthen your design. At a minimum, the application generally includes a summary of your design, detail about the protocol, a copy of data-collection forms, and the consent form. These must be developed and included with the application. Ask colleagues who are not intimately involved with your study to read your application and give you feedback on flow and consistency.

Table 5-1   Anatomy of an Informed Consent

Element	Contents
Purpose of the research project	• Presents a straightforward, clearly written explanation of the purpose of the study and why it is important • Describes why the individual was selected as a subject
Procedures	• Detailed explanation of what the subject can expect during the experiment • Comprehensive account of what will be expected of or done to the subject
Risks and discomforts	• Honest and comprehensive statements of risks that may be a result of the intervention or the lack of an intervention • Straightforward description of any discomfort—during or after the experiment—that the subject might experience
Benefits	• Description of any potential for direct or indirect benefit to the subject • If no benefit for the subject, contribution to the body of medical knowledge or patients in the future
Alternatives available	• Honest disclosure of alternative treatments available for the subject should they elect not to participate
Confidentiality	• A list of methods used to protect the information collected from the individual • Protections that will be put in place to assure that the subject and his or her responses will remain anonymous *(continues)*

Table 5-1   Anatomy of an Informed Consent (continued)

Element	Contents
Request for more information	• The name of an individual that the subject can contact for questions or for more information
Refusal or withdrawal	• Written assurance that the individual may refuse to participate without any consequences to them in the present or future • Notification of the right of the individual to withdraw from the study at any time, even after it has started
Treatment of injury	• Explanation of steps the subject can take to receive treatment for any negative effects attributable to the experiment
Consent statement	• Formal statement that the individual signs indicating that he or she is giving consent to participate

If you have ever presented a study at the IRB, you know that everyone is solemn, serious, and formal. For a novice bedside scientist, this may seem overwhelming. Preparation is the key to success. Try to get several team members to help present the details of the research plan. Do not be intimidated by questions; answer them to the best of your ability. If an answer is unknown, let the IRB know that you will find out and report back.

At least two IRB members will review each project in depth and make a recommendation to the full board. It is not unusual that revisions may be requested, or additional information solicited, before approval.

IRB-Exempt Review

Quality-improvement projects, with data used internally for quality improvement purposes, are often exempt from IRB review. The definition of exempt studies is very specific. It is still expected that the study will follow ethical standards, but full board review is not required. A summary of the project must be submitted, along with a Health Information Portability and Accountability Act (HIPAA) waiver explaining how patient confidentiality and anonymity will be preserved. Many survey designs and most qualitative studies are exempt from full IRB review. Check the guidelines for your IRB, as you must still submit information to the board, and you cannot proceed until the exempt status is documented. For example, a survey to evaluate nurse–physician communication would likely be exempt from full IRB review.

Expedited Review

In special cases, a study will have an expedited review process. Although the full review process can take a month or more, an expedited review is complete in a week or less. This type of review is most common when a low risk of harm and a high potential for benefit of a treatment exists. This is usually coupled with an urgent need for the treatment. For example, expedited review may be requested when a recent outbreak of a disease can be treated with the experimental intervention.

Compassionate Use

On rare occasions, a drug still under investigation may be used to try to preserve a patient's life when he or she does not meet study criteria. This may happen with patients who are in a critical state but do not meet the strict inclusion/exclusion criteria for a study that could benefit them. An example of this might be using a drug that was tested to destroy specific bacteria on a patient with a bacterial infection not targeted by the study.

NATIONAL INSTITUTES OF HEALTH GUIDELINES FOR RESEARCH ETHICS

The NIH has an entire branch dedicated solely to protection of both human and animal subjects in research. The NIH is a primary source of health care research funding through grants. Every proposed research project must have a section on protection of subjects; the ethics of research is infused throughout the entire grants proposal process.

In 2005, the NIH ruled that none of their investigators or any of their family members can have any affiliation with any company that might benefit from the results of a study they are doing. Under the NIH's guidance, all IRBs require that all primary investigators sign a yearly conflict of interest statement.

Strengthen Organizational Commitment to Your Research

Bedside science research projects are rarely successful without organizational support. Clinicians will need persistence, passion, and no small measure of frustration tolerance to navigate the organizational approval and resource allocation processes. Some ways exist, however, to improve your chances at successfully winning the support you need.

- Take time in a team meeting early in the process to brainstorm all of the possible stakeholders for your research project. Stakeholders include those that will be directly or indirectly affected by your study. Assign each stakeholder to a team member to discuss the study and get feedback about potential issues that can be addressed as design progresses.

- Find a champion among the leadership group early on. A leader champion can make sure that your study is considered for funding and formal organizational support. A champion in the leadership group can solicit support from others on the leadership team and "run interference" for you with other administrators.

- Solicit input from ethicists and IRB members before you finalize your application. Experienced members of the IRB can identify potential problems in your application and give you advice for improvement. An ethicist can help you strengthen the efforts that guard the rights of potential subjects.

- Take time to make accurate predictions of how much total time will be required for study preparation, recruiting subjects, applying the treatment protocol, and collecting data. Organizational leaders will want to know how many total salary dollars will be required as well as how much time is expected from staff. Consider nonsalary costs as well, such as postage for surveys, consultation with a statistician, specialized software or instrumentation, and other supplies and materials.

- Look for financial support from local and regional grant sources. Federal grants are often large and prestigious, but equally difficult to win. Many local and regional professional organizations award smaller grants, which may be sufficient for a focused bedside science project or a pilot study. The results of a pilot study funded by a local source may result in a larger grant for the full study awarded by a national organization.

- Learn your organization's budget cycle and request processes. Sometimes getting funds for a study is dependent on good timing and making appropriate written requests of leaders.

- Approach a local university to find graduate students who may be interested in helping with your project as part of a class requirement. New faculty may also be looking for a research agenda and may provide design and statistical support, in addition to helping with manuscript preparation.

The bar would be raised for all studies if researchers were required to evaluate each research project using the stringent guidelines of the NIH for grant funding. NIH guidelines are strict to assure that limited government funds are fairly distributed to scientists who are answering the most pressing questions and have the best designed ethical research studies. The NIH requires that we know what we should expect of ourselves as researchers. Although the project might be of limited scope, we should still be able to answer each of these questions affirmatively:

- Are we studying a pressing and important question?
- Are we focused and clear on what we plan to do?
- Do we have the right study methods, right team, adequate resources, and enough time?
- Is protection of the human subjects obvious?
- Is ethical treatment of everyone involved clearly demonstrated?

The NIH and IRB affect the ethical treatment of subjects and assure that other federal guidelines are met. Other legal requirements are imposed by the HIPAA and the Privacy Act of 1974 and are intended to assure that the patient's right to privacy of his or her medical information is protected.

SOME NOTES ABOUT HIPAA AND RESEARCH

Bedside scientists must meet the requirements of laws that are intended to protect the private medical information of patients in their studies. These laws apply to information that is collected directly from patients and indirectly from their records, even if the study is a small one. The two primary laws that affect the collection of medical information are the Privacy Act of 1974 and HIPAA. The Privacy Act was an early legislative attempt to control access to medical information but applied only to federally operated or funded health care facilities. HIPAA, which became effective in 2003, applies to all health care facilities and programs. The main thrust of HIPAA is to safeguard each patient's "protected health information" (PHI). Eighteen elements described in this law are considered protected, but the most common are the patient's name, social security number, medical history, diagnosis, and address. The social security number is specifically protected under the rule and cannot be used as an identifier except for claim submissions.

HIPAA changed the way every facility handles patient information and requires any facility providing direct patient care to publish a Notice of Privacy Practices. This notice must be given to all patients and informs the patient how his or her PHI will be used and protected. Patients can request an "accounting of disclosures," which informs the patient about anyone who had access to his or her records *without their express consent*. This means that all health care organizations must be careful about how they handle requests for patient information for research purposes. Because this legislation carries substantial monetary penalties for violation—such as using information without consent or divulging PHI to an unauthorized person—health care organizations scrutinize all requests for information that do not include the patient's express authorization or consent.

All organizations will require the researcher to obtain permission for access to data for any research activities, whether you collect the information directly from the patient or indirectly from their record. Check with your

Strengthen Your HIPAA Compliance

It may be tempting to avoid conducting bedside science projects for fear of violating HIPAA requirements. HIPAA was never intended to stop the progress of clinical research, but rather to provide an additional layer of protection for subjects and their health information. Several ways are available for you to accomplish your clinical research project and meet the requirements of the law:

• Obtain the patient's consent to use his or her information. This is the best way to gather information and comply with legal and ethical guidelines.

• Use deidentified data. Some facilities have limited data sets available or have the ability to strip identifiers from records before use.

• Use aggregate data. Data that are summarized at the unit, department, or organizational level do not represent individual cases and thus are not subject to HIPAA restrictions. You will still need organizational consent but will not have to file individual disclosure forms.

• Use data that were collected before April 14, 2003. According to the regulation, data existing before the implementation of the rule are not subject to the stricter HIPAA requirements, although these data are still subject to the Privacy Act of 1974. Check with your organization first, however. Some organizations made a decision to apply HIPAA requirements to all of their data, regardless of when it was collected.

• Use data on decedents. As a researcher, you will still be required to obtain permission from the organization, but generally, risk of disclosure for this type of data is not a concern.

organization's IRB or privacy officer to determine what the approval process involves. Be prepared to describe the information that you want to access, how it will be used and reported, and what measures you will take to ensure its security. This is required whether you are asking for decedent data, deidentified data, current information, or historical data. After receiving permission, you may be required to file a disclosure form in each record that you access for your research. These forms are used to keep track of access if the patient requests an accounting of disclosures.

You should never operate under the assumption that your research is exempt from the requirements of HIPAA or the Privacy Act. Even IRB-exempt research may still be subject to these legal requirements. Your research will proceed much more smoothly if you prepare your request for data access early in the process, determine the organizational protocols for approval, and follow the requirements conscientiously.

GETTING ORGANIZATIONAL COMMITMENT

Many legal and regulatory requirements must be met to start a study, but an awareness of economic and political considerations is necessary to finish it successfully. You will need to use all appropriate procedures to gain approval for your study and to get access to the subjects you need. These considerations are as important to the success of your study as meeting the regulatory requirements.

It is never too early to think about who you need to involve on your team to help gain commitment and support for your study. It is critical to give thought to all of the potential stakeholders in your study. Who will be directly affected by the study? Who will you need for support? Who can give you the resources that you need to carry out the research?

At the very least, consider who needs to know about your study and give their blessing for your study to be a success. If you plan to involve multiple disciplines, consider submitting this as a strategic initiative that is sponsored by a senior member of hospital management. Keep in mind the general equation that involvement equals commitment. By involving key stakeholders early in the planning stages, you can heed and address their concerns during design. Early involvement of those who will be affected by the study can avert many problems later in the process and can help you gain the help you need to make the study work.

As you develop your study plan, develop your resource plan as well. A flowsheet for managing and monitoring a bedside science project appears in

From the Mouths of Bedside Scientists: The Resources Clinicians Need for Practice-Based Research

What are some resources that you have discovered you needed as you conducted a bedside science research project?

Time. Time is always the most challenging resource. I do not know how often we thought we had the perfect study design, but when doing our pilot (let me stress here that you should always do a pilot—it will save significant heartache down the road), we realized that our enrollment process or data collection methods would take too much time to do realistically with our existing team. One of the studies that I helped pilot was just too time intense for our sick patients and their stressed families. We finally got rid of the patient questionnaire altogether and figured out other ways to get the most important data, rather than asking for it from the patients.

People and time. I had planned to do an orthopedic study but realized that I should have pulled a larger team together to help with the data collection. I eventually submitted the study as a grant and got funding for a research assistant to help with patient enrollment and data collection. When you are a busy clinician you should always involve others to partner with on research.

Expertise. Our team took over a year to try to figure out a way to do a study in our dialysis population. We did everything right but really were not sure about the study design. Then our hospital hired a PhD clinician who sat in on one meeting. "Voilà!" We were able to quickly bring it all together and submit it for IRB approval. It still would have taken us time to design our study, but in the future, we plan to include an experienced scientist with statistics expertise to guide us early on.

What resources were most important in making your study a success?

A good team and leadership support. We wanted to develop and study a rapid response team to decrease mortality and length of stay. We had senior management support and key individuals from trauma, the intensive care unit, and the hospitalist program, which included nurses, physicians, respiratory therapists, pharmacists, and an experienced clinician–scientist. Because of the team and the leadership support for this hospital-wide effort, we got the research support that we needed to design a neat project. We also got data collection support, which allowed clinicians to do what they do best—take care of the patient.

Money. Think about getting a grant for your research project. Even small grants help. Good research takes time. A grant is tough, but it helps you focus on all of the resources (time, costs, individuals, etc.) that you need to do your study well. I think I designed a better study for a diabetes clinic outcomes project because I had to submit a grant.

Appendix 5. An early economic analysis will help you quantify the necessary resources. Be sure to consider all of the resources that you may need, including staff time, supplies, expert consultation, and money. A pilot study can be invaluable in testing the procedures on a small group and can give you more accurate estimates of the resources that will be needed.

Communicate the research design and resource plan using appropriate channels. One way for organizational commitment of research to grow is for senior management to understand that the resources that are needed for studies will have a positive impact on patient outcomes.

For more depth and detail, try these resources:

Center for Medicare/Medicaid Services information about HIPAA: www.cms.hhs.gov/hipaa.

CFR (Code of Federal Regulations) 164.501, 164.508, 164.512 (i) [HIPAA Law].

Ecoffey, C., and B. Dalens. 2003. Informed consent for children. *Current Opinion in Anaesthesiology* 16: 205–8.

Foster, C. 2001. *The Ethics of Medical Research on Humans.* London: Cambridge University Press.

Kamienski, M. 2000. Tips on navigating your research proposal through the Institutional Review Board. *Journal of Emergency Nursing* 26: 178–81.

O'Herrin, J.K., N. Fost, and K.A. Kudsk. 2004. Health Insurance Portability Accountability Act (HIPAA) Regulations: Effect on Medical Record Research. *Annals of Surgery* 239: 772–8.

Olsen, D.P. 2003. HIPAA Privacy Regulations and Nursing Research. *Nursing Research* 52: 344–8.

Portney, L.G., and M.P. Watkins. 2000. *Foundations of Clinical Research: Applications to Practice,* 2nd ed. Upper Saddle River, NJ: Prentice Hall.

Shamoo, A.E., and D.B. Resnik. 2002. *Responsible Conduct of Research.* London: Oxford University Press.

Silverman, H.J., J.M. Luce, P.N. Lanken, A.H. Morris, A.L. Harabin, C.F. Oldmixon, B.T. Thompson, and G.R. Bernard. 2005. Recommendations for informed consent forms for critical care clinical trials. *Critical Care Medicine* 33: 867–88.

WHERE TO FIND THE RESOURCES YOU NEED

Many resources in our clinical environment go untapped because they do not have the name "research" associated with them. Check with your *quality department* for statisticians, data experts, analysts, access to data warehouses, and project management support. *Organizational and staff development* will likely have project management experts, consultants skilled in focus groups, help with qualitative research methods, and support for training related to your protocol. The *medical library* can help with literature searches and access to databases. In larger organizations, *management engineering*

Table 5-2   Resource Needs for a Bedside Science Project

Research need	Internal Hospital Resources	External Community Resources
Research idea	Your colleagues Journals Patient-practice issues Quality department Human resources	University librarian Academic teachers and clinical instructors Newspapers and magazines Conferences and symposia
Literature review support	Medical librarian Your colleagues	University librarian Academic teachers
Study design and analysis	Quality department analysts Management engineering Doctoral-trained clinicians Clinician researcher with statistics expertise Medical residency program Biostatistician Organizational development or marketing department (for survey development)	Partnership with colleges or universities Biostatistician consultant

may provide research support relating to workflow, process improvement, and high-level culture-change projects. *Environmental safety* usually has access to industrial engineers who have a strong understanding of study methods. *Marketing departments* are often repositories of rich population level data and information related to satisfaction and complaints.

As a researcher, you will always have resource limitations. No bedside scientist gets all of the time, money, and support needed to complete a project. Creative partnerships throughout your organization can be beneficial. Create opportunities for networking within your organization. Professional networks can both help you find the right people for a project and gain their support.

Table 5-2   Resource Needs for a Bedside Science Project *(continued)*

Research need	Internal Hospital Resources	External Community Resources
Data access and collection	Health information management department Quality department Infection control Human resources Residents Nurses on light duty	External grants to fund data collectors Students
Reports, abstracts and publications, posters and presentations	Staff Medical Editor Clinician-Researcher with publishing experience and expertise Media services Marketing Secretary with PowerPoint skills	Professional copy centers
Practice change	Protocol committee Unit leaders Leadership committees(s) Clinician researcher	Professional organizations—collaboration with other members

SUMMARY

Do not underestimate the importance of organizational commitment to the success of your research project. Identify stakeholders early in the process and involve them in its planning. Organizational support and access depend on your ability to address legal, ethical, political, and economic realities in your project plan. Organizational resources may be spread throughout your organization; thus, take the time to look for help even if your organization does not have a research department.

Legal considerations for the researcher include those presented by HIPAA; make sure your plan is HIPAA compliant. Prepare the IRB application carefully. The IRB review may take the form of a full board review, an exempt project, expedited review, or a compassionate use project. Use NIH guidelines to assure that the study is well designed, considers carefully the rights of subjects, and has a positive risk–benefit analysis. Considering all of these elements—in addition to the scientific merit of the study—can enhance the chances of a successful bedside scientist study.

Part III

Designing the Structure of a Bedside Science Project

Design, Study Methods, and Procedures

You have been reading research about the care of neonatal skin and have come across an article that is counter to the results you have already read. Although most of the current research indicates that using alcohol on a neonate's cord does more harm than good, this study seems to indicate that alcohol is better at preventing infection. You look for other explanations for the finding—and you do not have to look far. After looking over their charts and doing a physical exam, the researcher personally picked the subjects for the sample. If objective criteria were used, you cannot find them. Maybe they biased the treatment group? You cannot figure out the procedure that was used on each group to care for their cord. Although the researcher states that measures were objective and reliable, no supporting statistics are provided for this statement—such as measures of interrater reliability—and the measures appear to be subjective, including descriptive phrases such as "degree of redness" and "smell of infection." You are not entirely sure that it is an experi-

mental design because you have no way of knowing how subjects were assigned to groups. You hesitate to be too critical, as you are new at this systematic review process; maybe it is your fault that you cannot figure out the procedures that were used. After all, it was published, albeit in a little known journal. While reading the fine print, you see that a company that makes alcohol swabs sponsored the study. On seeing this, you put aside your doubts about your critical abilities and toss the journal article in the "poor-quality" pile. You are not convinced that there are not a lot of alternative explanations for the link between the treatment and the outcomes in this study, and the alcohol swabs do not seem to be the primary explanation—at least not a strong enough explanation to ignore the pile of good studies that you have indicating that alcohol is not the best for neonatal cords.

A good methods section serves several purposes in a research article. First, the methods section should present an accurate and thorough account of every important step in the design and conduct of the research. This thorough account allows the reader to make decisions about accepting the results of the study. Providing sufficient detail about the methods used in the study enables the reader to decide for himself or herself how much confidence he or she has that the experimental treatment did indeed lead to the results. Second, a strong methods section supports replication—one of the hallmarks of sound research that contributes to an overall professional body of knowledge. In practical terms, you should be able to conduct the study exactly as the author did, using your own subjects, to determine whether the results can be generalized to another population. Finally, a thorough methods section allows a comparison of findings across studies. This is critical for the systematic review process. A thorough account of the subjects, intervention, measurement, and analysis allows for a comparison across studies to draw conclusions about both the size of the treatment effect and the consistency with which outcomes are achieved.

This section of a research study is the basis for your conclusions about the validity of the findings. Your critical appraisal of study methods should lead you to the conclusion that inconsistency in *procedures* is not an explanation for the results. In other words, can you exclude all other rival explanations for the outcome, except that of the intervention? If the methods section is sound, the answer to this question should be an unequivocal "yes," giving you the confidence to apply the findings to your own practice.

The methods section is relatively standard; a good methods section will review the sampling strategy, the design of the study, instruments, procedures, and analysis. Although length limitations imposed by journals may limit the depth of detail that an author can provide, you should be able to determine the key elements to assess its validity. A valid study is one in which all other variables have been controlled so that the effect of the experimental treatment can be isolated. This is no small task and is one that is essential for the application of evidence in practice.

INTERNAL VALIDITY

If we are to feel confident incorporating a new treatment into our practice based on research, then we have to be sure that the treatment was the only variable that led to the outcome. A study that effectively isolates treatment effects from confounding ones is considered internally valid. Common threats to validity are bias and unexplained variability. Three main sources of bias and variability exist: the researcher, the procedures, and the subjects. A detailed description of threats to validity and associated controls appears in Table 6-1.

Each threat presents challenges to the validity of a study and each requires specific strategies to assure control.

Researcher Bias and Variability

Human nature leads a researcher to have some preconceived ideas about how a research study will come out. If the researcher did not believe that a treatment is effective, the effort to test it would not be expended. Nevertheless, this very belief in the effectiveness of a treatment can lead to a form of bias—researcher bias—that may affect the outcome. Although most researchers would not consciously "set up" an experiment to achieve a predetermined result, unconscious or subconscious motives exhibit themselves as a host of threats to validity.

The most common manifestation of researcher bias is selection bias. Consciously or unconsciously, the researcher may either select subjects or assign subjects to groups based on some criteria that are not objective. When criteria are not objective, then a subject may potentially be assigned to the experimental group because he or she has characteristics that might prove the researcher's point or conversely assigned to the control group because he or she is more likely to have a bad outcome.

For example, a researcher may be testing a procedure to speed healing of wounds and select subjects from a pool of orthopedic subjects. Without objective selection, there is a possibility that patients with very small wounds might be mixed in with patients with large, suppurative wounds. The patients might

Table 6-1   Common Threats to Internal Validity and Associated Control Measures

Threat	What It Is	How It Is Controlled
History	Events occur during the study that have an influence on the outcome of the study.	Random sampling to distribute effects across all groups
Reactivity/ Hawthorne effect/testing effects	Subject reactions that are due to the effect of being observed	Unobtrusive measures Subject blinding The use of sham procedures or placebos
Instrumentation	Influence on the outcome from the measurement itself, not the intervention	Calibration of instruments Documentation of reliability Analysis of interrater reliability
Maturation	Effects of the passage of time	Match subjects for age Use analysis of covariance to measure effects of time
Regression	Extreme values gravitate toward average if repeatedly measured, regardless of the intervention.	Use reliable instruments Random sample to minimize extreme values
Attrition/ experimental mortality	Subject attrition is caused by dropouts, loss of contact, or death.	Project expected attrition and oversample Carefully screen subjects before recruitment Thorough consent procedures so that subjects are aware of what will be expected of them

Table 6-1   Common Threats to Internal Validity and Associated Control Measures *(continued)*

Threat	What It Is	How It Is Controlled
Bias	Study is influenced by preconceived notions of the researcher or reactions of the subject.	Blinding of researcher, data collectors, and subjects as to who is getting the experimental treatment
Confounding variables	Variables affect the outcome but are not primary variables being studied.	Randomization to distribute effects of variables Use of analysis of covariance to measure the effect of confounders
Treatment diffusion	Members of the experimental group do not get the whole treatment, or members of the control group get some of the treatment.	Isolate experimental subjects from control subjects Careful protocols for application of the treatment
Statistical conclusions	Inaccurate inferences are drawn because of inadequate power or violation of statistical assumptions.	Adequate sample sizes Prospective calculation of power Test for violation of assumptions before analysis
Selection	Subjects are assigned to groups in a way that does not distribute characteristics evenly across both groups.	Random selection Random assignment Matching of subjects Stratified samples

be in varying degrees of nutritional deficiency and may be of very different ages. Patients with co-morbid problems that inhibit healing—such as diabetes, or smoking—might be mixed in with those who have a singular, simple diagnosis. Without objective criteria, we cannot be sure that wounds that heal faster are due to the treatment and not to the patient's nutritional status, age, or the effects of other diseases. It might not be a problem to have this range of diversity in a subject pool if the subjects are assigned to groups randomly. Bias is most evident, however, when subjects are assigned to groups other than randomly, with the potential for "stacking the deck" in the experimental group. Without random assignment, it is possible that improved results may be due to something other than the treatment.

Random assignment assures that most alternative explanations—called extraneous variables—are evenly distributed between the experimental and the control group. Without random assignment, the researcher might (quite unconsciously) put the sicker, older, less nourished patients with multiple co-morbidities all into the control group, virtually assuring that they will have a harder time healing. If healthy, young, well-nourished individuals are primarily in the experimental group, they are nearly guaranteed to have speedier healing. Objective selection and random assignment are critical to controlling selection bias. These aspects are so important to good design that Chapter 7 of this book is dedicated to subject recruitment, selection, and assignment processes, collectively called the sampling strategy.

Although selection bias is probably the most common form of researcher bias, the individual who is most vested in a research study may affect the outcome in a multitude of ways. The critical reader will search for signs that a researcher affected the outcome—through the selection of instruments, training of observers, and analysis of the data—in order to exclude a possible link between the outcome and the actions of the researcher. Another common way to control research bias is blinding. When a study is blinded, the researcher does not know which subjects are in the experimental group and which are in the control group. This eliminates the potential for a researcher to affect the outcome of the study by consciously or unconsciously manipulating the results of the experiment.

The methods section should report clear measures and procedures that have been selected appropriately, tested rigorously, applied reliably, and recorded accurately. These characteristics should apply equally to the application of the treatment and to the measurement of the outcome. If you cannot understand the specific procedures that were used or if you find them confusing, do not blame your own critical abilities; the researcher's obligation is to spell them out in a way that is both thorough and understandable.

From the Mouths of Bedside Scientists: How Clinicians Talk About Design

What makes a measurement reliable?

When I think of the word *reliable*, I also think of *consistent*. When I am using an automated blood pressure device, each time I use it on the same patient, using the same size blood pressure cuff that is placed on the same spot on the arm, it gives me the same reading. You will notice that I describe several specific steps that need to happen to make the measurement consistent. A caution exists, however. When I think of reliable, I sometimes want to make assumptions that reliable means accurate, honest, true, and so on. It does not. It only means consistent. You could be consistently right, consistently almost right, or even consistently wrong. As with many statistics terms, you can only take it for what it means and not assume anything else.

What kind of bias have you had to guard against?

Bias is the reason I am so careful about how I design a study. I look at advertisements on television and know immediately that producers are trying to bias me toward using their product. However, I know that facts are what I want to know before I will even consider buying a product. In the same sense, every time I have done a study I know that I need to think about bias. I know that I always need to watch for ways that my team and I may inadvertently influence what we hope to see happen.

I think believing in something and bias goes hand in hand. As a clinician scientist, I have realized that my beliefs can, in fact, be a detriment to what I am trying to study. Thus, I engage my colleagues to help keep me honest and "unbiased" in my study designs. As much as possible, I try to do studies in which both the patient and I are blinded to the intervention. I have a greater challenge in studies where I know one patient is getting a treatment and another is not.

Why are experimental designs better to support evidence-based practice changes?

I have always heard how experimental designs are the "gold standard" to support evidence-based practice. Now that I have begun doing research myself, I am beginning to understand much better why that is. It is because those results are much less likely to have been influenced by bias or chance. It means that you can trust these findings as being real and as "standing up" in your environment as well. Perhaps "levels of evidence" should in fact be called "levels of reduced bias" because the better the evidence, the less likely that the results are biased.

Procedures: The Treatment

In an experiment intended to test a treatment, the researcher should clearly identify and describe the experimental intervention. This intervention is called the independent variable, called such because it is not a naturally occurring element in the situation under study. Often referred to as a "manipulation," it is a critical part of the study. In order to be confident that a given outcome was a result of the intervention, the treatment has to be applied to the experimental group consistently. Otherwise, *variations* in the treatment could be the cause of the outcome instead of the treatment itself; carefully controlled treatments strengthen the validity of a study.

Where to Look for Information About the Methods and Procedures

- The methods section is generally identified in a straightforward way and labeled "methods." It is occasionally called "research design" or "plan." Other words may appear in the heading, such as *methods and procedures* or *methods and materials*.
- This should be easily identifiable and is a major part of the research study write-up. The description may be concise, but should have enough detail that an informed reader could replicate the study.
- If the intervention or measurement is complex, there may be a separate section for procedures, which may be labeled as such, or called "protocols." This section may describe either the specific steps for applying the treatment or for measuring its effects (or both).
- What is *included* in the methods section is *not* always standard. The section should have subheadings for the sampling strategy, research design, treatment protocols, measurement, and analytic plan.
- The measures may be called "instrumentation" or "tests." If a survey is used, a separate section may describe the development of the instrument, as well as procedures for its completion by subjects. Information about reliability and validity should be provided with the description of the instrument.
- It is not unusual to find that the author describes the instrument rather than providing a copy; this is not a weakness. The survey may be copyrighted or proprietary, or limitations on the length of the article may preclude its inclusion.

Labeled "protocols," "treatment," or "plan," the specific procedures for the treatment should be laid out in detail. Timing, duration, and frequency of implementation should all be described. A reader should be able to reconstruct specific procedures for the intervention from the description. Clear, written protocols will help support the objective and reliable application of the treatment. The more clarity there is in the directions, the greater the probability that variations in treatment can be excluded as a cause of the outcome.

It is not enough to have clear procedures, however. If the *researcher* is applying the treatment, the chance of a researcher bias effect increases. As a result, researchers often use individuals to implement the treatments who are not directly associated with the study. These individuals bring objectivity to the experimental intervention, but can also introduce variability of their own if they are not adequately trained and monitored. A thorough intervention plan includes control of the treatment through a clear protocol, training plans, and steps to assure the protocol is implemented the same each time it is applied. The same controls should be in place for each step of the experiment, including the measurement systems and data collection procedures.

Measuring the Outcome

Clarity in specification of the outcome is as important as a clear description of the treatment. The outcome is referred to as the dependent variable, because its occurrence is dependent on an intervention (or, in the case of the control group, lack of an intervention.) Capturing the effect of an independent variable on a dependent variable requires careful specification of the outcome, as well as the selection of a measurement instrument that can detect the outcome when it occurs.

Dependent variables may be measured in many ways. A researcher may use an instrument to capture a physical response—such as a radiologic exam, calipers, or laboratory measures. Computer software programs, observation, interviews, or surveys may be used to record patient history, health status, risk factors, or psychosocial responses. Examples include the Functional Independence Measure, the Faces Pain Scale, or the Short Form 36 for physical functionality.

The dependent variable may be measured via primary data collection methods, meaning that the measurements are taken directly from subjects in the study. For example, if a pharmacist is interested in studying medication reactions, a report of signs and symptoms of adverse events may be solicited directly from patients. The dependent variable may also be measured using secondary data collection. Secondary data are retrieved from the recordings made by others. If the pharmacist used secondary data, evidence of drug reactions might be recorded directly from the patient record.

Primary data may seem superior but nevertheless have limitations. Primary data are time consuming to collect, and the quality of the data depends on many factors. The patient's recall of a physical reaction or an event may be quite different than reality. Some subjects may not be able to communicate clearly, or language barriers may be present that distort reporting. The individual taking the recording may not use consistent questions, language, or approach. Inflection may lead a patient to "the answer that is wanted," a version of treatment effect. For example, the question "do you abuse alcohol?" will elicit a far different response than "how many alcoholic drinks do you consume in a week?" The response to either can be affected by the tone of voice of the questioner. Those doing the data recording must be carefully trained in data collection techniques. The consistency of data captured by multiple raters must be checked by measures of interrater reliability.

Secondary data are often easier and quicker to collect. Particularly in organizations that have made great progress toward an electronic patient record, patient-level data may be retrievable. Ease of access is limited by the organization's procedures for research approval and assurance that HIPAA standards are being met; answering specific research questions generally requires a moderate level of skill at writing computer requests and using search engines.

Even if the organization does not have an electronic medical record, additional resources are available for secondary data collection. Many hospitals have cost accounting systems that store rich data related to volumes of both patients and procedures. Some cost accounting systems also contain proxy measures of patient severity and productivity, such as the capture of relative value units. Additional sources of secondary data are decision support systems—generally residing in the information technology or health information management departments—that allow for answering a complex array of research questions. The quality department also has access to data that are extremely helpful for research, such as trends, quality indicators, improvements, and their results.

Sources of publicly available aggregate data exist, such as the Centers for Disease Control, the census bureau, or the Healthy Persons 2010 database. Various data registries (such as the US Renal Dialysis Data Set) provide data for a fee. State hospital associations and public health departments have a broad range of data available for evaluating the health of populations and the distribution of disease.

Secondary data collection has its limitations as well. The accuracy and completeness of the data are dependent on the individuals capturing and recording the data. Physician notes, nursing notes, collaborative plans, and teaching plans are only as thorough as the author. Gaps in information may mean either a re-

For more depth and detail, try these resources:

Anstey, K.J., and S.M. Hofer. 2004. Longitudinal designs, methods and analysis in psychiatric research. *Australian and New Zealand Journal of Psychiatry* 38: 93–105.

Bale, S. 2004. Using different designs in wound healing research. *Nurse Researcher* 11: 42–54.

Bellini, J.L., and P.D. Rumrill. 1999. Validity in rehabilitation research. *Journal of Vocational Rehabilitation* 13: 131–8.

Boissel, J. 2005. Planning of clinical trials. *Journal of Internal Medicine Supplement* 742, 257: 36–48.

Fitzgerald, S.M., P.D. Rumrill, and J.D. Schenker. 2004. Correlational designs in rehabilitation research. *Journal of Vocational Rehabilitation* 20: 143–50.

Henson, R.K. 2001. Understanding internal consistency reliability estimates: A conceptual primer on coefficient alpha. *Measurement and Evaluation in Counseling and Development* 34: 177–89.

Hulley, S.B., S.R. Cummings, W.S. Browner, D. Grady, N. Hearst, and T.B. Newman. 2001. *Designing Clinical Research,* 2nd ed. Philadelphia: Lippincott, Williams, and Wilkins.

Kurpius, S.E., and M.E. Stafford. 2005. *Testing and Measurement: A User-Friendly Guide.* Thousand Oaks, CA: Sage Publications.

Morgan, G.A., J.A. Gliner, and R.J. Harmon. 1999. Evaluating the validity of a research study. *Journal of the American Academy of Child and Adolescent Psychiatry* 38: 480–6.

Portney, L.G., and M.P. Watkins. 2000. *Foundations of Clinical Research: Applications to Practice,* 2nd ed. Upper Saddle River, NJ: Prentice Hall.

Schulz, K.F., and D.A. Grimes. 2002. Case-control studies: Research in reverse. *The Lancet* 359: 431–4.

sponse did not occur—or the clinician simply did not record it. Data retrieved from secondary sources that are paper—such as many patient records—provide two sources of potential data error. The data may not be recorded correctly from the primary source, and the individual retrieving the data from the chart may miss it or record it inaccurately.

The more automated the data collection systems for a research project, the better the chance that the data will be complete and accurate. If, on the other hand, no solid secondary source exists for data, the researcher may need to use instruments to collect primary data directly from subjects.

Instrumentation

Instruments are used to measure variables directly from subjects. The primary concern with physical instruments (e.g., thermometers) is calibration. Keeping instruments in top working condition and well calibrated minimizes measurement error. Not all instruments are easily calibrated, however. For example, how do you calibrate an instrument to measure stress? In the case of instruments that measure characteristics or traits, the calibration concern is replaced with an emphasis on reliability and validity.

Reliability: A Focus on Consistency

Instruments are considered reliable if they consistently measure a given trait with precision. When a measure is reproducible, that is, when it generates nearly the same value every time it is used appropriately, it is considered precise. When a measure is precise, then the reader has a level of confidence that differences between groups are not explained by differences in the way the trait was measured. Reliability tells you that an instrument is stable within the instrument, across individuals, and over time.

These three types of stability can be tested statistically and should be reported with the description of the instruments. Stability within an instrument is called internal reliability and is measured with the alpha coefficient statistic. This coefficient may be called Cronbach's alpha, coefficient alpha, or internal reliability and should have a value of 0.7 or greater. Stability between individuals is measured by an item–total correlation, which should have a positive sign and an absolute value that is close to 0.5. Stability over time is quantified by a test–retest correlation coefficient of 0.5 or greater. At least one test of reliability should be performed and reported for instruments used in an experiment.

A specific type of reliability assessment is indicated when multiple raters observe and record a variable. Interrater reliability quantifies the stability of a measure across *raters*. For example, the degree of agreement between two or more physical therapists who are measuring range of motion should be documented. A simple percent agreement can be used to document interrater reliability, but a kappa statistic is even better. Specifically called Cohen's kappa, this statistic focuses on the degree of agreement between raters and generates a p value, reflecting the statistical significance of the agreement. A kappa can be interpreted like a percentage, and in either case (percent agreement or kappa), a value of 0.85 or greater is considered acceptable. An associated small p value indicates that the agreement was not due to chance. A high kappa (> 0.85) with a low p value (< 0.05) reflects good reliability between multiple raters in an experiment.

If the instrument is researcher developed, it should be pilot tested on a small group of subjects for assessment of reliability. These pilot tests should be performed and reported as part of the methods.

Another Way to Look at Reliability

A measurement instrument must be reliable before it can be valid. In other words, a measurement instrument must be consistent before we can determine whether it measures what it is supposed to measure. Even widely accepted measurement tools may be unreliable if they are not used or maintained properly.

An example is my bathroom scale. Like most people I know who are my age, I get on my bathroom scales with some trepidation—I do not always like what I see. I have found, however, that if I lean back on my heels, I can lose 3 pounds! If I simultaneously rest my hand lightly on the towel bar, I can lose up to 5 pounds. In fact, my husband now tells me if I want him to lose weight I am going to have to install a sturdier towel bar.

Now, when I lean back on my heels and rest my hand on the towel bar, have I really lost 5 pounds? Unfortunately, no. The procedure that I am using for weighing myself is not consistent, and therefore, the answer will not be consistent. Because it is not consistent, it will not reflect my actual weight.

The measurement you get when using an instrument is called the observed score and the actual value of what is being measured is called the true score. When the observed score consistently reflects the true score, then we say the measure is reliable and valid. On the other hand, if the observed score consistently overestimates or underestimates the true score, then the measure can be neither reliable nor valid. When I am weighing myself—to be truthful—I would just as soon have an instrument that consistently underestimates the true score. In virtually every research study, however, we would prefer that the measurement instrument consistently measures the subject's attributes accurately.

Validity: Accuracy and Truth

An instrument has to be reliable to be precise, but a measure can be consistently wrong. For example, it is difficult to measure the length of a neonate. The child is measured from the heel to the crown of the head—not exactly a precise description. Thus, measuring over the head to the tip of the nose would be more reliable; it is easy to find the end of the nose, but it would not be an accurate representation of the baby's length. Reliability tells us an instrument will be consistent; validity tells us the instrument will consistently measure the right thing.

Validity is harder to test than reliability. For example, you are familiar with the faces pain scale—a scale of 10 visual faces, with the lowest end a smile and

Table 6-2   Reliability and Validity Tests: Meaning and Interpretation

Test	What It Means	Interpretation
Cronbach's alpha/ coefficient alpha	Internal reliability; are the individual items consistent with the overall test results?	Coefficient alpha should exceed 0.7 as a minimum; below 0.4 is unacceptable; 0.4 to 0.7 is weak reliability; 0.7 to 0.9 is moderate reliability; > 0.9 is strong reliability
Guttman split half/ split half alpha	Internal reliability; is the first half of the test as reliable as the second half, or, are odd numbered items as reliable as even number items?	Split half will be lower than coefficient alpha, but should exceed 0.6 as a minimum
Parallel reliability	Is the instrument as reliable as an instrument that is similar in intent and content?	Yields a correlation coefficient, which should exceed 0.5
Test–retest reliability	Is the instrument stable over time? If used repeatedly, are the results due to actual changes in the subject, not the instrument?	Yields a correlation coefficient, which should exceed 0.4
Face validity	Does the instrument look like it measures the concepts it is supposed to?	No statistics; generally reported as expert review or agreement
Criterion-related validity	Does the instrument measure actual performance or presence of the characteristic it is intended to measure?	Correlation coefficient of greater than 0.7
Interrater reliability	Do two or more raters agree on the ratings?	Percent agreement of 0.85 or greater; Cohen's Kappa of 0.80 or greater with a p value less than 0.05

the upper end a face with a frown and tears. How do we know the upper icon does not represent depression to the subject and not pain? Thus, although there are several ways to measure and report validity, it is still a difficult undertaking. Table 6-2 summarizes some of the most common tests of reliability and validity and a guide for their interpretation. It is not uncommon to see reliability reported with no measure of validity.

However, there *are* several ways to document validity. *Content validity* involves a subjective judgment about whether a measurement makes sense.

Hitting the Stacks

Collins, Kershaw, and Brockington used a randomized control trial to determine whether oral nutritional supplements, delivered by community nurses, could improve nutritional status and wound healing in home-nursed older persons. "Subjects were randomized into the two supplement groups in a block design using random numbers. Both groups received routine wound care, usual nursing care, and the daily nutritional supplement. Each subject was provided with a 4-week supply of supplement (28 cans) and encouraged to consume 80 ml three times a day, with meals. The two supplements were in indistinguishable cans. The study was double blinded, with the subject and the research nurse unaware of the supplement allocation group. . . . At week 4 the number of cans of supplement consumed by each subject was recorded."

Sethares and Elliott evaluated the effect of a customized message intervention on, among other things, beliefs about the benefits of and barriers to compliance with diet and medication. These concepts are sometimes difficult to measure reliably, but the authors found and documented a tool with acceptable psychometric qualities. "Internal consistencies of the Beliefs about Diet Compliance Scale and the Beliefs about Medication Compliance Scale were psychometrically evaluated in a convenience sample of 101 clients with heart failure. Internal consistencies of these 2 subscales were found to be 0.87 for benefits of medication, 0.91 for barriers to medications, 0.84 for benefits of diet, and 0.69 for barriers of diet. Content validity of the tool was found when evaluated by 2 heart failure experts, with 81% agreement on the content."

Collins, C., J. Kershaw, and S. Brockington. 2005. Effect of nutritional supplements on wound healing in home-nursed elderly: A randomized trial. *Nutrition* 21: 147–55.

Sethares, K., and K. Elliott. 2004. The effect of a tailored message intervention on heart failure readmission rates, quality of life, and benefit and barrier beliefs in persons with heart failure. *Heart and Lung* 33: 249–60.

Content validity can mean that face validity has been assessed ("this instrument *looks like* it should measure pain") or that a panel of experts has verified that the correct concepts are included in the measure. *Construct validity* indicates that a measurement conforms to accepted theoretical standards. There are many types of *criterion-related validity*, which is the correlation of the instrument to some external manifestation of the characteristic. Criterion-related validity can be concurrent, when an instrument reflects actual performance. An example might be when the reading from an aural thermometer is correlated with the reading from a rectal thermometer. Criterion-related validity might also be predictive, indicating that a measure can predict future performance, or demonstrate the capacity to differentiate those who have a characteristic from those who do not.

Most validity tests use the correlation coefficient to represent the degree of relationship between the instrument and the reference. Unlike reliability, when a 0.7 is considered the cutoff for acceptability, it is uncommon for a validity coefficient to be greater than 0.5. The seminal works of Cohen established the standard for effect size of a validity coefficient: < 0.2 = weak; 0.21 to 0.4 = moderate; > 0.5 = strong.

Considerations in Instrument Selection

At a minimum, calibration and/or internal reliability should be reported for any instruments used in the experiment. The study becomes stronger as more documentation of the reliability and validity of the instrument are provided. The tests and their actual results should be reported and jointly are called the "psychometric properties" of the instrument.

It is not uncommon to use instruments that are borderline acceptable statistically. There are many considerations in instrument use in addition to the reliability and validity properties. Feasibility of administration, costs of instruments, and the type of measures considered professionally acceptable also drive the selection of an instrument. Acceptability for the subject is a strong consideration. It might be more accurate to use urine collected before dawn because it is more concentrated, but it is not acceptable to wake a patient at 4 a.m. to solicit a urine sample. The acceptability of a treatment and a measure can affect patient responses and attrition of study subjects.

Variation Caused by Subjects

Subjects themselves provide variation in an experiment. There is some intrinsic variability in applied health care studies because people are different, and the way they respond to treatments will vary from individual to individual. Although a careful sampling strategy can minimize the effects of individual variability, not all error can be controlled with sampling.

A strong threat in an experiment is the patient's *belief* about the treatment and about being a subject in an experiment. The fact of observing a subject often changes the subject's behavior. This phenomenon was observed in early experiments called the Hawthorne studies and thus is often referred to as the Hawthorne effect. In the Hawthorne studies, subjects in a factory changed their behavior regardless of the intervention that was applied because they knew they were in a study and tried to please the researchers. This can be an extremely common occurrence in health care, where patients feel helpless and dependent on clinicians. In experiments with discernible treatments, this may also be called the placebo effect.

Blinding may also be used to control subject effects. If the subject is unaware whether they are receiving a legitimate treatment or a placebo, then treatment effects are equalized between groups. This is most easily accomplished in drug trials, when a sugar pill may look identical to the real drug. This approach is not limited to drug trials, however; a subject in a control group may get a sham treatment that resembles an actual intervention but is not therapeutic. For example, in a study of the effect of acupuncture on the nausea of pregnancy, one group received acupuncture applied at therapeutic sites, whereas the control group received acupuncture at random sites. In this study, the researchers were able to isolate the effects of therapeutic needle insertion from the placebo effect of needle insertion in general.

Diffusion of the treatment, sometimes called contamination, may occur in experiments where it is difficult to withhold the intervention from a control group. For example, it may be difficult to ask a control group to completely avoid exercise or to sleep only 4 hours a night. In the early experiments seeking treatments for HIV, subjects in experiments would sometimes trade half of their medications, so desperate for treatment that they concluded that getting half of a dose (or double) was better than the risk of being in the control group. Contamination threatens the validity of an experiment, particularly if no significant differences are found. Are there no differences because the intervention had no effect, or did some of the control group also get the intervention?

Validity is threatened when subjects leave an experiment before the experiment is finished. Longitudinal experiments, or experiments over time, are particularly vulnerable to attrition of subjects. Subjects may move, drop out, or become unavailable. Sometimes called "mortality" in experiments, attrition may literally be due to patients dying during the experiment. A certain level of attrition is expected; in good studies, attrition is compensated for with a sound sampling strategy. As long as attrition is random, it is generally not problematic. Systematic attrition, or attrition because of a shared characteristic, may weaken a study. A group that could contribute information is lost. For example, if a measurement instrument requires reading, systematic attrition may include all of those who are illiterate or for whom English is a second language.

Many threats to the validity of an experiment exist. A good experiment is one in which the treatment has an effect on the outcome and all other effects have been excluded. The researcher may have bias that affects the experiment. The procedures and instruments may also introduce unexplained variability. The subjects may contribute sources of error. To a certain extent, a sound sampling strategy (explained in depth in Chapter 7) can control many threats to validity. Fundamental control, however, is achieved through a combination of a good research question that is linked to the appropriate research design.

RESEARCH DESIGN

The choice of a research design is dependent primarily on the question that has to be answered. Research questions fall into three general groups. A research question may seek to *describe* a phenomenon or population. It may

Strengthen Your Studies

It is difficult to conduct a pure experimental design in an applied setting. Extraneous variables abound, and it is often unethical to withhold treatment from a control group. It is hard to assure that the experimental group always gets the treatment exactly the same. Time constraints and availability of individuals to collect data can hinder the validity of the experiment. Although it may be challenging to conduct a true experiment in a working unit, there are still measures you can take to strengthen the validity of your studies:

- Use a comparison group of some kind. Although it may be difficult to assign patients to groups randomly, the use of a comparison group does strengthen validity, even if it is a convenience sample.

- If using a nonrandom comparison group, match the groups as closely as possible on potential extraneous variables, such as age, severity of illness, number of co-morbid conditions, etc.

- A common method of obtaining a comparison group is to measure a baseline in a group of subjects and then repeat the measure as the treatment is applied. This design—called a repeated measure design—has a great deal of power. The baseline can be considered a comparison group.

- Clearly identify your independent and dependent variables and write formal operational definitions of each. These definitions can help you determine criteria for inclusion in the study, treatment protocols, and measurement systems.

have as a goal the study of *relationships* between variables or between subjects, or it may lead to the investigation of *differences between groups*, such as in a true experiment.

Descriptive Studies

Many research questions set out to describe the characteristics of a group of subjects. A researcher may be interested in the rate of adverse drug reactions in a specific ethnic group or the level of anxiety in preoperative children or the needs of families in a waiting room. For these types of research questions, a descriptive research design is appropriate. Descriptive designs may involve random sampling based on selection criteria, and any variety of measurement instruments—from surveys to observations to calibrated hardware—may be used. Reports of results generally include tables, graphs, and visual representa-

---

Strengthen Your Studies *(continued)*

- Use simple, straightforward measurement methods whenever possible. Measure unobtrusively to minimize treatment effects.
- Take advantage of automated systems to capture data whenever possible, including the recording systems that are built into some patient care equipment, such as intravenous pumps, automated beds, and medication administration systems.
- If you are using a chart review to capture data, select a random sample of charts to limit the labor involved in data retrieval.
- Training is critical. Train those who will apply the treatment and those who will collect the data. Set up monitoring systems and random checks to assure that the treatment and measurement systems are working consistently.
- Hide the identity of the experimental and control groups from those who are collecting data whenever possible. Blinding of those who are both subjects and data collectors minimizes several threats to validity, including treatment effects and researcher bias.
- Get help when designing your study. Individuals in your quality department, members of the medical staff, and people in a research department can help you talk through your design and identify areas where it could be strengthened.
- Replicate the studies of others whenever possible. Finding a study that reports an experiment similar to yours can help jump start your study by describing procedures and measures that you might be able to use.

tions of data. Descriptive studies do not yield p values because the researcher is not looking for differences or associations, and thus, measures of sampling error are not relevant.

Correlation and Prediction

Many consider correlation and prediction studies to be primarily descriptive. These studies are appropriate for research questions that ask about relationships between variables or between subjects. When an actual association is measured, the study is called a correlation study. A correlation study may answer a question about the nature and strength of a relationship between two variables in the same subjects (is there an association between emergency department visits and incidence of depression in patients with chronic obstructive pulmonary disease?) or between two subjects on the same variables (is there an association between age of onset of menopause in mothers and daughters?). A correlation coefficient is used to analyze the relationship. Although still considered descriptive, a correlation coefficient does yield a p value, which represents whether the relationship is due to sampling error.

A cautionary note is warranted, however, about the use of statistical significance in evaluating correlations. A correlation simply describes the nature and strength of a relationship—not cause and effect. Confounding variables may explain the relationship, or the variables may simply share some logical trait. For example, a correlation exists between eating ice cream and swimming accidents. Do we believe that ice cream causes swimming accidents? Of course not. Both events occur more frequently in the summer and thus would have a strong correlation, even though no causation is implied by the relationship.

A second type of correlation uses regression techniques to determine whether one variable can predict another. A more sophisticated type of descriptive statistic, regression design, is useful when a research question focuses on whether the incidence of one variable can be used to predict the values of another variable. For example, given a patient's total cholesterol, could the level of cardiac risk be predicted? Regression designs also yield a p value, which allows for the testing of hypotheses about the relationship, and an r-squared statistic, which quantifies how much variation in the outcome can be predicted. These statistics will be described in more detail in Chapter 8.

Descriptive, correlation, and predictive studies all involve the collection of variables from a group of subjects or secondary data sets. None of these designs, however, will measure cause and effect. Causal relationships are demonstrated by a group of designs that reflect true experiments.

Experimental Designs

Experimental and quasiexperimental designs allow for tests of differences between groups that are due to some causal event. In a true experiment, subjects are randomly assigned to an experimental group (that receives a treatment) or a control group (that does not.) If validity is controlled, differences between groups are considered attributable to the intervention, called a treatment effect.

True experiments are the strongest designs for drawing conclusions about causal relationships. The randomized controlled trial is considered the strongest experimental design for measuring cause and effect. In a randomized controlled trial, subjects are randomly assigned to either an experimental group (that receives an intervention) or a control group (that receives no intervention or a standard intervention). Randomized controlled trials are rated as the highest level of evidence in a systematic review and the only designs from which cause and effect can be appropriately inferred.

In order to determine cause, three conditions must be met: the cause must precede the effect; the cause must demonstrate an influence on the effect; and rival explanations must be excluded. The controls provided by a true experiment meet all three conditions.

True experimental designs are not easy to conduct, however. Finding adequate samples, randomization, and instrumentation may provide significant barriers. Sometimes it is not ethical to withhold the treatment from a control group, or it may be impossible to manipulate the independent variable. For example, it may be unethical to withhold a comfort measure from a patient or to limit educational materials for patients. Some independent variables cannot be manipulated, such as eye color or intelligence, and some should not be manipulated, such as error-free medication administration or skin care. In these cases, limitations lead the researcher to a design that controls as many extraneous variables as possible so that validity is maximized.

Experiments in which subjects cannot be assigned or randomized to groups are called quasiexperimental designs. Although not as strong in evaluating causal relationships as experimental designs, quasiexperimental designs can still provide good information about treatment. Quasiexperimental designs make use of comparison groups, but the element of randomness is not possible. The comparison group may be a group that asks for no treatment. It may be an intact group, such as patients on a unit that uses one type of hand cleaner compared with a unit that does not. Comparison studies may involve finding individuals with the independent variable naturally occurring—such as hypotension—and comparing them with a group in which the variable does not occur. This latter type of study is also called ex post facto, case control, or causal comparative.

Regardless of the type of study, the researcher should provide a clear link between the research question and the rationale for the selection of the design. The design provides control for validity and enables the researcher to draw accurate conclusions about the variables under study.

SUMMARY

The primary purpose of the methods section is to lay out clearly the variables under study, the procedures and measures used to determine results, and the means for controlling the validity of the study. Sufficient detail should be provided so that the reader could replicate the study with reasonable effort. The primary question the critical reader should ask is whether alternative explanations could have caused the results described in the study. These alternative explanations may be due to the researcher's bias, the procedures used, the measurement instruments, or the subjects themselves. Good studies have a clear link between the research method and the design. Designs may be descriptive, correlative, experimental, or quasiexperimental, and the rationale for selection of the design should be explicit. Assuring validity in a research study ensures the reader that he or she can be confident that the findings are appropriate to apply to his or her own practice.

Concepts in Action

A randomized controlled trial is considered the "gold standard" of research and contributes to level I evidence, the highest level of evidence for clinical practice. This design controls many sources of bias in an experiment so that the effects of an intervention can be isolated and quantified. Bedside scientists read and use randomized trials to determine the effectiveness of clinical interventions, and thus, familiarity with their unique characteristics is a critical understanding. With this in mind, pay careful attention to the study components unique to a randomized controlled trial as you review the following example, including use of a control group, randomization, blinding, and calculation of sample size.

What were the questions studied in this bedside science project?

Do two types of topical anesthetics—one of which takes effect faster than the other—work equally well in controlling the pain and anxiety associated with pediatric venipuncture? Can topical anesthesia work in both nonurgent and urgent situations?

Concepts in Action *(continued)*

Why was this research question important?

Needle sticks are frequent and necessary aspects of pediatric hospital care. Unfortunately, even a brief painful procedure such as a blood draw can result in significant pain and distress for a child. For venipuncture, subcutaneous injection with local anesthetic may be helpful, but it requires another needle stick and may produce pain on infusion of the anesthetic. Children who have difficulty coping with venipuncture are likely to be equally distressed by the local anesthetic infiltration. Clinicians at this academic community hospital on the East Coast continually searched for the best method of providing effective topical anesthesia that is painless, fast acting, and effective in controlling pain. It was expected that the child's anxiety level would also be decreased if the pain associated with venipuncture was avoided.

Topical anesthetics usually consist of a concentrated form of anesthetic that can be absorbed through the skin. Anesthetic is applied to normal intact skin for a certain length of time (usually an hour or more) to allow the skin at the application site to become numb. This numb area means that the pain from a needle puncture procedure is significantly minimized and often eliminated. Topical anesthetics deaden the nerve endings in the skin. They do not cause unconsciousness as do general anesthetics used for surgery, and they do not require the monitoring that would be necessary with forms of sedation. As such, they are a desirable alternative to venipuncture alone if effective.

These products vary in their ingredients, time to effect, and risk of complications. The two topical anesthetics compared in this project were Food and Drug Administration–approved medications for the age group and indications identified in this project. The first—EMLA—requires 60 minutes to achieve effectiveness and can have a vasoconstrictive effect. The alternative topical anesthetic—LMX4, formerly Ela-Max—requires only 30 minutes to reach effectiveness and does not cause vasoconstriction.

If all of the clinical and behavioral outcomes appear equal between the two topical anesthetics, the shorter time to effective local anesthetic in pediatric patients and the lack of a vasoconstrictive effect will be strong reasons to prefer one drug over the other. For nonurgent patients, this result can be directly applied to practice. A second question, answered by studying children with an urgent need for venipuncture, compares a duration of application that is shorter than 30 minutes to no topical

(continues)

Concepts in Action *(continued)*

anesthetic at all (placebo). In the part of the study focused on urgent patients, if the agent provides superior clinical and behavioral outcomes compared with no therapy, this will also be a strong reason to initiate the use of this drug in that patient population, even if for less than 30 minutes.

Who was involved on the research team?

This was a multidisciplinary project team led by a pediatrician and a pediatric pharmacist. Team members included several experienced pediatric nurses, an emergency department nurse research coordinator, and other clinical and research experts.

What were the methods that were planned?

Subjects were recruited from inpatients and outpatients at the medical center and met the criteria described in Table 6-3.

Table 6-3   Inclusion and Exclusion Criteria for EMLA/LMX4 Study

Inclusion Criteria	Exclusion Criteria
Patients meet each of the following criteria. 1. Children ages 5 to 18 years of age 2. Treated as an inpatient or outpatient within the past 24 hours 3. Venipuncture order, which is their initial venipuncture order 4. Are in one of the following groups: • Urgent venipuncture or blood draw, that is, must have labs drawn less than 30 minutes *and can wait at least 15 minutes for the blood draw* • Nonurgent venipuncture or blood draw, that is, able to wait at least 60 minutes for lab draw	Patients have none of the following criteria. 1. Known allergy to EMLA, LMX4, or any of their ingredients 2. Known sensitivities to local anesthetics of the amide type, lidocaine, or prilocaine 3. Multiple abrasions or injuries that affect both hands 4. Brain injured or disoriented (Glasgow Coma Scale < 15) 5. Cognitively impaired (Mini Mental State Examination < 28) 6. History of skin conditions, including one or more of the following: a. Frequent skin rashes b. Eczema c. Unexplained bruising

Concepts in Action *(continued)*

The study design and procedures were based on a study by Koh (1999), and thus, Koh's data were used to calculate power. For a power of 80%, with an acceptable alpha of 0.05, 43 subjects were needed in each group.

After recruitment and consent, patients were assigned to one of two parts of the study based on urgency of venipuncture or lab draw. The first part of the study consisted of those patients requiring nonurgent venipuncture who could wait at least 60 minutes to have the procedure. The second part of the study consists of those patients requiring urgent venipuncture (less than 30 minutes) but who were able to wait at least 15 minutes for the procedure. These patients would normally not be candidates for topical anesthetic due to the urgency of their status. On enrollment in the nonurgent part of the study, patients were randomly assigned to one of two topical anesthetics: LMX4 or EMLA. On enrollment in the urgent arm of the study, the patients were randomly assigned to one of two groups: LMX4 or placebo.

After the patient is assigned to a group, a standard *procedure* for the topical anesthetic was used: A study nurse applied the topical anesthetic to both antecubital fossa and the back of both of the child's hands. An occlusive covering—provided in the study pack—was applied over the topical anesthetic.

In the nonurgent part of the study, the drug was left in place 60 minutes (for EMLA) or 30 minutes (for LMX4). In the urgent part of the study, LMX4 or placebo was in place for 15 minutes under occlusive dressing.

After the topical anesthetic was applied, a questionnaire was administered to obtain anticipatory anxiety ratings from both parent and child. Ten minutes before the venipuncture, children were brought to a procedure room. A nurse began observing signs of behavioral distress immediately after the child entered the room. Parents and children in both experimental groups were encouraged to do what they would typically do to cope in the situation. An age-appropriate book was left on the procedure table for parents as a possible means of distraction for the child. After the venipuncture, the child was asked by the nurse to rate the pain that was experienced.

Measures included the child's report of pain and observed behavioral distress. Pain ratings were obtained after the venipuncture, with the child rating the amount of pain experienced during the venipuncture using the Wong-Baker FACES Pain Rating Scale (Figure 6-1). This scale asks the child to rate pain from no pain at all to "hurts worst"—the worst pain ever

(continues)

Wong-Baker FACES Pain Rating Scale

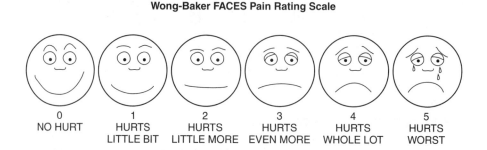

0	1	2	3	4	5
NO HURT	HURTS LITTLE BIT	HURTS LITTLE MORE	HURTS EVEN MORE	HURTS WHOLE LOT	HURTS WORST

Figure 6-1   The Wong-Baker FACES Pain Rating Scale. *Source:* **From Hockenberry, M.J., Wilson, D., & Winkelstein, M.L. (2005). Wong's essentials of pediatric nursing (7th ed., p. 1259). St. Louis, MO: Mosby. Used with permission. Copyright © Mosby.**

Concepts in Action *(continued)*

(Wong & Baker, 1991). Three behavioral distress ratings were recorded on a 6-point numerical scale (0 = not at all distressed; 5 = extremely distressed) by one of two nurses. The ratings were obtained for time periods described as (1) anticipatory, behavior from treatment room entry until the tourniquet was placed; (2) insertion, the behavior at the time of the needle stick; and (3) recovery, behavior after venipuncture. A score of 0 was assigned if the patient had no sign (verbal or physical) of distress and cooperated with the venipuncture. A score of 5 was assigned if the patient was hysterical and required significant physical restraint to do the venipuncture. Scores in between represent distress levels between these two extremes. A second researcher independently rated behavioral distress for approximately a third of the subjects, and interrater reliability was checked.

All pediatric project personnel were trained in the use of the behavioral distress scale before collecting data.

Children were asked to rate their levels of anxiety about having venipuncture. This was measured with a 100-mm vertical visual analogue scale ("using this scale, please tell us how anxious you are about having venipuncture"), with anchors of "not nervous at all" and "extremely nervous." At the same time, parents or guardians rated the degree of their own anxiety about their child having venipuncture by completing a similar 100-mm visual analogue scale ("using this scale, please tell us how anxious you are about your child having venipuncture").

In both parts of the study, children rated their anxiety as the nurse prepped them for venipuncture and again after the venipuncture, both

Concepts in Action *(continued)*

times using the 100-mm visual analogue scale. The last evaluation assessed how anxious they were about the venipuncture.

Previous Needle Stick Experience

Parents or guardians were asked for (1) the number of needle sticks (blood sampling, IV placements, and immunizations) that their child had experienced in the last 2 years and (2) their child's level of difficulty coping with these previous sticks on a 100-mm visual analogue scale (anchors of "not at all difficult" to "extremely difficult").

Difficulty of Venipuncture

The nurse who did the venipuncture answered a series of questions rating the degree of difficulty (100-mm visual analogue scale) in locating a suitable vein for venipuncture and the venipuncture itself.

What were the challenges that were faced?

This project was challenging to complete because many of the patients thought to meet study criteria had to be excluded. The planned timeline for the study appears in Figure 6-2. Even with this level of planning, a lack of time and adequate resources was a barrier. It took almost 2 hours to complete the study procedures once a patient was enrolled. A busy pediatric or emergency department staff nurse had to enroll the patient. This was not an externally funded study, and thus, funded projects had priority over this one. Also, during the course of the study, there were significant leadership changes on the general pediatric unit that had an impact on this study.

In light of these challenges and because during the study time period additional evidence emerged that showed the equivalency of EMLA versus LMX4 use in pediatric patients, the nonurgent part of the study was closed early. This enabled a focus of resources on the urgent part of the study. The urgent part of the study—which sought completely new knowledge about the procedure—continued as planned. Locations for subject recruitment were expanded so that additional subjects were available and additional support was available in the urgent part of the study.

How was this study used?

As a result of this study, awareness of the qualities and uses of both EMLA and LMX4 has increased and both are now used; before the

(continues)

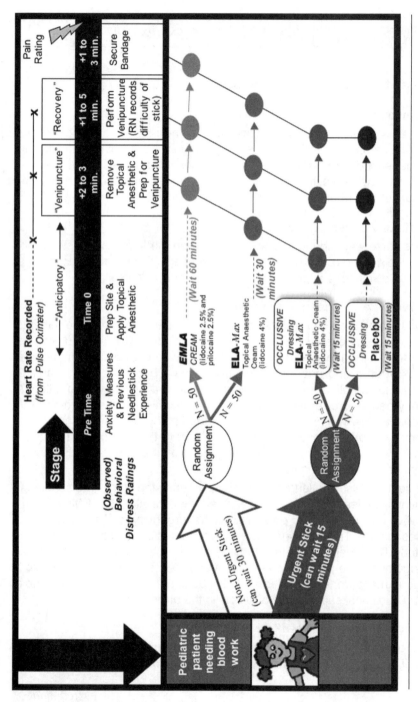

Figure 6-2   Planned timeline for the EMLA/LMX4 study.

Concepts in Action *(continued)*

study, EMLA was the primary topical anesthetic used. It is expected that after the study is complete, LMX4 will be used under occlusion in all urgent venipuncture sticks that can wait at least 15 minutes.

How it will be communicated internally and to larger audiences?

This study is shared internally in multidisciplinary monthly reports and in staff meetings. Publication in a peer-reviewed journal is expected, as the primary body of the manuscript has been written. It will also be shared as a poster or presentation at a pediatric conference and at regional research conferences.

Koh, L., D. Fanurik, M. Schmitz, and M. VonLanthen. 1999. Efficacy of parental application of eutectic mixture of local anesthetics for intravenous insertion. *Pediatrics* 103: 79–83.

Checklist for Evaluating the Methods and Procedures of a Research Article

_____ The design is clearly identified.

_____ A rationale is provided for the choice of a design and it is linked to the research question.

_____ A specific procedure is described for the application of the treatment or intervention.

_____ Instruments and measures are described objectively.

_____ Reliability of the instrumentation is described, and supporting statistics are provided.

_____ Validity of the instrumentation is described, and supporting statistics are provided.

_____ A detailed protocol for the use of each instrument in the measurement is described.

_____ Threats to internal validity are identified and controlled.

_____ Researcher bias and treatment effects are controlled by blinding.

CHAPTER 7

Sampling Strategy

In this chapter, you will learn to

- Evaluate the way a sample is selected
- Determine whether the sample size is adequate
- Decide whether study findings apply to your population
- Select the best sample that you can for your experiment

Your critical care unit is interested in determining whether an open visiting policy affects patient outcomes. As a critical care nurse, you are convinced that open visiting interferes with patient care, but you promise yourself that you will stay objective and open minded throughout the experiment. It is convenient and easy to access your own unit; thus, your research team asks to measure outcomes under the existing restricted visiting policy and then change to an open visiting policy and measure again. Your plan is approved, but you decide to wait to initiate the project until the work is a bit slower on the unit. Data are collected for 4 weeks, and then open visiting is initiated. It is difficult to collect the data consistently, as flu season hits just as your unit initiates open visiting; nevertheless, you feel confident that you have captured the data accurately. After the research is completed, the research shows that patient outcomes were better under a more restrictive policy. When you present your findings to your clinical policy group, you call for a policy that restricts visiting in all of the critical care units. You are quite surprised when you are greeted with a less than enthusiastic

> *response. The sampling strategy is criticized as "potentially biased and not representative" and is cited as the reason for not immediately adopting your recommendations. "What do these people want," you think, "I've given them the evidence that they need to implement these findings, and they are just not listening!"*

Sampling strategy is a critical part of research design but is one that is rarely executed well. In fact, the sampling plan is often one of the weakest aspects of research studies. An adequate sampling plan is critical for the application of findings to other people, settings, or time periods. Nevertheless, many published and applied research studies are based on convenience samples that are too small to provide a conclusive test of the research question. It is common to focus on design, measurement, and analysis—even when the use of an inadequate sample virtually eliminates the possibility of applying the findings in a broader way.

That is not to say that every member of a target population needs to be included in every study. It is rarely practical (or even possible) to include every potential subject in a study. Most research studies use a subgroup—a sample—to draw conclusions about a larger group—a population. Although *using* a sample for research is common and appropriate, the way the sample is chosen (known as the *sampling strategy*) has broad implications for how you *apply* the research results. The most important questions that you have to answer when evaluating a research sample are those that affect whether the sample is *biased* and whether the results can be *generalized*. The questions that guide your evaluation of the sampling strategy include the following:

- Were the subjects selected in an objective and consistent way?
- Were enough subjects included to be comfortable with the conclusions?
- Do the subjects that were studied reflect the patients in my practice setting?

Ultimately, the sampling strategy will be the primary determinant of whether the results of a study are valid and whether they can be generalized to a larger and/or different group. When evaluating research for quality, two primary elements should be looked for: selection strategy and sample size. *The ideal sample has objective selection criteria, is randomly assigned to groups, and has achieved at least 80% power.* The authors should report these elements of the sampling strategy in clear, straightforward terms in the methods section of a research article.

SELECTION STRATEGY: HOW WERE THE SUBJECTS CHOSEN?

Selection strategy is a primary way of controlling bias in a research study. *Selection bias* occurs when a researcher has an effect on the subjects selected for the experiment and/or the assignment of subjects to groups. Selection bias may be conscious but is more commonly unconscious and is of particular concern when the researcher has preconceived ideas about how the study will turn out.

Inadequate sampling can also lead to *sampling bias*. A biased sample underrepresents or overrepresents some characteristic in the sample. Unfortunately, samples that are easiest to recruit may introduce sampling bias into a study. For example, subjects that are recruited primarily from a tertiary-care center may inherently include more serious patients. Conversely, recruiting from outpatient settings may underrepresent the severity of a condition. Sampling bias increases *sampling error* as well as the chance that the researcher will draw misleading conclusions.

Even with a rigorous sampling plan, certain segments of the population may refuse to participate or be unable to participate. Sampling bias may be present when a group is *too* homogeneous so that it does not reflect the diversity in a population. A homogeneous sample makes generalizing to other populations difficult. Historically, samples for medical research have been heavily weighted with white males. In the past decade, researchers have been more sensitive to the need for a broad representation of ethnic and gender groups in research, but gaps in representation still exist.

Another kind of selection bias occurs when subjects elect *not* to participate. Systematic sampling error can occur when response rates are low or attrition is high. There are many reasons that subjects may decline to participate in a study or may drop out after it has started. A certain amount of refusal and/or nonresponse is to be expected in any study. However, the researcher should describe the reasons for refusal or attrition in order to assure that systematic sampling error is not exhibited. For example, if all of the individuals who refuse to participate are from a particular ethnic group, socioeconomic status, or educational level, then the final sample is not representing the entire population.

CONTROL OF BIAS IN SAMPLING

Three aspects of sampling strategy can control bias. These controls include the development of objective selection criteria, sound methods for recruitment of subjects, and the use of probability in sample selection or group assignment.

Selection criteria may involve inclusion criteria, exclusion criteria, or both. The use of *inclusion criteria* provides guidelines for choosing subjects with a predetermined set of characteristics. The author should clearly outline inclusion criteria for the study, and you should be able to find these criteria where the sample is discussed. These criteria define the major factors that are important to the research question and may include clinical, demographic, geo-

From the Mouths of Bedside Scientists: How Clinicians Talk About Sampling

Why sample?

There is something about defining a sample that helps me better define my research question and study. It is just as reliable (if you sample correctly) as what the entire population could tell you, and it is much more feasible to do. There is *no way* I could use an entire population!

What does a random sample mean?

This means that I will get a "representative" group of individuals that reflects characteristics of the entire population.

What does random assignment mean?

This means an individual has just as much chance of being in the group that is the experiment as in the group without an experiment.

What is a type II error?

When you sadly feel like your study is for naught . . . when you should have looked a little more carefully at the way you determined your sample size—you might have seen that your intervention did in fact make a difference. (That one fact alone has taught me to work more closely with our biostatistician and to learn more about statistics—yikes—myself!)

graphic, and temporal criteria as appropriate. The primary function of inclusion criteria is to limit the potential for selection bias by objectively identifying who can be considered a subject.

Many authors also include *exclusion criteria*, or characteristics that exclude a potential subject from the study. Some individuals are not suitable for the study, even though they meet the inclusion criteria. These subjects might have clinical exclusion criteria (e.g., co-morbid conditions that might affect the study) or behavioral exclusion criteria (e.g., high likelihood of being lost to follow-up). Exclusion criteria fulfill the same function as inclusion criteria and help to control extraneous variables.

The method of recruiting subjects should be clearly identified. Although the ideal sample is randomly drawn from a known population, it is a nearly impossible feat to accomplish. Not only is a list of the total population rarely available (e.g., how would you get a list of all people with hypertension?), but

Where to Look for Information About the Sample

- Look for a description of the sampling strategy in the methods section. It may be labeled *sample, subjects,* or *participants.*
- A description of the *characteristics* of the sample will likely appear in the results section. If the researcher has conducted statistical tests of group equivalency, the results of those tests should appear here. This is to demonstrate that the experimental and control groups have roughly the same characteristics. You are looking for test results that show no differences between groups. In other words, tests for group equivalency should *not* be statistically significant.
- You may not find a description of the sampling strategy. This is particularly true if a convenience sample has been used. If you cannot find a description, it is safe to assume that the sample was not selected randomly and is a convenience sample.
- The words *probability sample* and *random sample* mean the same thing. Conversely, the words *nonprobability sample* indicate that the sample was one of convenience.
- It is common that specific calculation of power is not reported. This is not a problem if the results are statistically significant—if results are significant, then the sample had adequate power (even if the sample was small.) If results are *not* statistically significant, then reporting of power calculation is essential to avoid a type II error. You cannot assume that negative results are conclusive without a calculated power of at least 80% (0.80). Because power can be calculated retrospectively, there is no reason *not* to report it.

most researchers do not have unlimited access to the population. A sample that is drawn carefully will "look like" the population and can be used to draw conclusions about the larger group, even when the entire population cannot be included. The only way to be sure that a sample represents a population is if it incorporates an element of randomness.

The best studies have samples that are either randomly selected or randomly assigned to experimental groups. A researcher might have no choice but to ask accessible subjects to join the study and thus potentially introduce bias. If the researcher randomly assigns the subjects to experimental groups, however, then any differences between the sample and the population are evenly spread out over all groups in the experiment.

THE GOLD STANDARD: THE RANDOM SAMPLE

Random in research does not mean that the researcher just picks any number. "Random" is actually a mathematical concept. A random sample is one that meets two criteria: every member of the population has an equal probability of being selected for the sample, and the selection of a member is an independent event. The first criterion is one that allows us to assume that the sample represents the population. If every member has an equal probability of selection, then a random sample will represent the diversity as well as the similarities in a population. This random selection process can be carried out in several different ways.

Simple Random Sampling

Simple random sampling is when a table of random numbers (either computer generated or from a textbook) is used to select subjects from a list of the entire population.

Systematic Random Sampling

Systematic random sampling is useful when the researcher is unsure how many individuals will eventually be in the population. It is a practical way to draw a sample from a prospective group, that is, a group that is in the future. In systematic random sampling, the first subject is drawn randomly, and remaining subjects are selected at predetermined intervals.

Stratified Random Sampling

Stratified random samples are structured so that important characteristics are evenly distributed across all groups. The researcher first divides the population into groups based on some characteristic (e.g., gender, ethnicity, and diagnosis) and then picks a representative sample from each group.

Cluster Random Sampling

Sometimes it is impossible to draw single subjects from groups, either because of geographic limitations or accessibility issues. In cluster sampling, the researcher randomly selects entire groups and then randomly selects subjects from only those groups.

The second criterion—independence—is more of a statistical concern than one of representation. Independence is violated if we get more than one score from the same subject. The most common nonindependent sample is a pretest/posttest. Time-series data, or data collected on the same sample over

---

Hitting the Stacks

Buchanan et al. (2004) use well-defined inclusion and exclusion criteria for their exploratory study of an intervention for tobacco dependency. "Inclusion criteria were: adults 19 and older who (a) smoked 10 or more cigarettes per day, (b) had access to a telephone, (c) lived within driving distance, (d) were in preparation or action stage, (e) were willing to use nicotine replacement therapy (NRT), (f) had no contraindications to NRT use, and (g) had a primary care provider. Exclusion criteria were: active cancer, nicotine sensitivity, untreated cardiovascular disease, or unstable condition that would interfere with participation in the study."

Stout et al. used both criteria and power calculation to strengthen their study of an intervention to reduce pain in emergency department patients during lumbar puncture. "Based on an alpha level of .05 and a power of 80%, power analysis determined a sample of 45 subjects in each of 2 groups (N = 90) would detect a difference between groups in pain scores. . . . Patients were considered for inclusion if a lumbar puncture was planned in the emergency department and they were able to give informed consent. Other criteria for study inclusion were age 18 years or older; ability to read, write, and speak English; and ability to use the numeric rating pain scale. Exclusion criteria included allergy or sensitivity to lidocaine; indwelling electrical device (pacemaker or insulin pump); conscious sedation per hospital policy; and rash, skin break, or scarring over the selected site."

Buchanan, L.M., M. El-Banna, A. White, S. Moses, C. Sidelik, and M. Wood. 2004. An exploratory study of multicomponent treatment intervention for tobacco dependency. *Journal of Nursing Scholarship* 36: 324–30.

Stout, T.D., A.A. Schultz, M.R. Baumann, P.J. Jordan, B. Worthing, and J.H. Burton. 2004. Reducing pain in ED patients during lumbar puncture: the efficacy and feasibility of iontophoresis, collaborative approach. *Journal of Emergency Nursing* 30: 423–30.

---

time, are also nonindependent. When data are not independent, then we know that the score on one measure shares some characteristics with the score on another measure. A researcher can compensate for nonindependence with specific statistical tests, but the nonindependent nature of the data has to be recognized and dealt with.

THE MORE COMMON SAMPLE: CONVENIENCE SAMPLING

When random sampling is not realistic, then the researcher often relies on *convenience sampling*. Convenience sampling—as it sounds—is based on subjects that are accessible to the researcher. Obvious advantages exist for us-

---

Strengthen Your Samples

It is likely that you will have to use convenience samples for bedside science studies—they are the subjects accessible to you. You can strengthen a convenience sample by taking some simple steps, however:

- Develop inclusion and exclusion criteria, and apply them consistently. This will lower the risk of selection bias.
- Use an element of randomness. Although you may not be able to select your sample randomly, you can randomly assign subjects to an intervention or control group. The process does not have to be complicated—flipping a coin or rolling dice are both acceptable methods of randomization.
- Conduct a power calculation so that you know that you have an adequate sample size. Use the automatic power calculator located at http://www.powercalc/ucla to determine how many subjects you need to detect differences. If it is not possible to prospectively identify sample size, use the power calculator to determine how much power you did have in your sample, particularly if you did not find anything significant.

---

ing convenience sampling, primarily logistics and cost. Keep in mind that convenience sampling can introduce bias into the sample. Selection bias might be present if the researcher is involved in personally selecting the subjects. Consciously or unconsciously, the researcher's predetermined ideas about the research might affect subject inclusion.

A specific kind of convenience sample that violates both randomness and independence is *snowball* or *referral sampling*. In snowball sampling, each subject is asked to recruit other subjects. Although this may be the only way to reach some groups (e.g., alcoholics, drug addicts, or family members), the subjects are not independent and randomly selected, and thus, generalizing the results may be limited.

Convenience sampling is often used in pilot studies, when the specifics of a research study have yet to be determined. A small study conducted with a convenience sample can help determine the specifics of a larger study. In this situation, convenience sampling is acceptable and expected.

Even in pilot studies, however, when convenience sampling is necessary, then the researchers should do as much as possible to limit the bias that is inherent in this sampling method. The best way to reduce bias in a convenience sample is to assign subjects randomly to groups after they have been recruited.

For more depth and detail, try these resources:
Fredman, L., S. Tennstedt, K. Smyth, J. Kasper, B. Miller, T. Fristsch, M. Watson, and E. Harris, 2004. Practice and internal validity issues in sampling in caregiver studies. *Journal of Aging and Health* 16: 175–302.
Hulley, S.B., S.R. Cummings, and W.S. Browner. 2001. *Designing Clinical Research: An Epidemiological Approach*, 2nd ed. Philadelphia: Lippincott, Williams and Wilkins.
Melnyk, B., and E. Fineout-Overholt. 2004. *Evidence-Based Practice in Nursing and Healthcare: A Guide to Best Practice*. Philadelphia: Lippincott, Williams and Wilkins.
Minke, K., and S. Haynes. 2003. Sampling issues. Chapter in *Understanding Research in Clinical and Counseling Psychology*. Mahwah, NJ: Lawrence Erlbaum.
Spring, M., J. Westermeyer, L. Halcon, K. Savik, C. Robertson, D. Johnson, J. Butcher, and J. Jaranson. 2003. Sampling in difficult to access refugee and immigrant communities. *Journal of Nervous and Mental Disease* 191: 813–19.
Williamson, G. 2003. Misrepresenting random sampling? A systematic review of research papers in the Journal of Advanced Nursing. *Journal of Advanced Nursing* 44: 278–88.

Keep in mind that populations and samples are not restricted to human beings. "Subjects" might refer to documents (such as medical records), counties, or patient care units. In a particular kind of evidence-based research called meta-analysis, the "subjects" are actually research studies. Regardless of the unit of analysis, the sample should be selected based on preset criteria, and the best samples are selected with some element of randomness.

SAMPLE SIZE AND POWER: HOW MANY SUBJECTS ARE IN THE SAMPLE?

While subject selection determines whether the results can be generalized to a larger population, the number of subjects in the sample affects whether the results can be trusted. In general, sample size is the primary driver of the *power* of a sample. Adequate power means that there are enough subjects to detect a difference. The calculation of power is a mathematical process and may be calculated prospectively (to determine how many subjects are needed) or retrospectively (to determine how much power a sample possessed.)

Another Way to Look At It

Power is an interesting concept in that its effects are most apparent when you *do not* find anything in a research study. Inadequate power means there were not enough subjects in the sample to find what you were looking for (if it was indeed there.) Thus, it can be a real problem—were the results insignificant because there is truly nothing to be found, or was it there and we just could not find it?

An example can help us understand power. My husband is a big guy—he is about 6 foot 3 inches and more than 200 pounds. That does not mean, however, that he is fearless; in fact, he is terrified of spiders. If he has to go into the shed after dark, he always asks me to "sweep the shed for spiders" and let him know whether it is safe to enter. Suppose that the only light I can find it a 4-inch flashlight running on a couple of old AA batteries—not much illumination. If I look around the shed with the little, dim flashlight and do not see any spiders, how comfortable do you think my husband is that there really are not any spiders there? Not very comfortable—meaning that whatever chore he needed tools for is not going to get done.

On the other hand, what if I use his preferred method for spider sighting—a generator hooked to a 4-foot spotlight? If I check the inside of the shed with that amount of power going to the light, and I do not see any spiders, do you think that he is more comfortable going in there? If I use a great deal more power to check for spiders and I say there are none there, then I am more likely to get my leaky faucet fixed before dawn.

Think of a sample as a source of illumination. When a great deal of power exists in a sample, you can see the differences and relationships that are there. If you do not find anything with a powerful sample, then it is very likely that it is not there. However, when you do not have much power in a sample—when the sample is small—then you cannot be as comfortable saying that there was not anything there to begin with. Thus, we worry most about power when the results *are not* significant. *Of course, if you find something (even with a small sample), then you had enough power. It is only a problem when you do not.*

If power is insufficient, then a type II error is more common. A type II error occurs when there is a difference between groups, but the researcher does not detect it. In other words, the intervention works but the researchers do not conclude that it does. Power is primarily a function of sample size, and thus, inadequate samples are most suspicious when results are *not* significant.

In general, larger samples are more desirable from many perspectives. Larger samples have more power and less sampling error. Larger samples are more likely to be normally distributed (to fall in a bell curve), which is an assumption of many statistical tests.

A note is in order about very large samples, however. When samples get very large, then standard error (the basis for statistical significance) gets very small. When standard error is very small, then even inconsequential differences between groups may be statistically significant. Statistical significance only assures us that a difference is *real*, not that it is *clinically important*. This is a particularly important consideration in very large samples.

SUMMARY

Sampling strategy is critical for application of research findings to larger or different populations. Selection criteria and an element of randomness can assure that selection bias is minimized and representation is maximized. Sample size is an important consideration in power, or the ability to detect differences using a sample. The sampling strategy should be clearly described and is the basis for trusting the results and applying them to your patients.

Concepts in Action

Have you considered a bedside science project but felt overwhelmed by the amount of time it might take? That is when you can be grateful for the concept of "sampling." Sampling lets you complete a study with efficiency, maximizing information while minimizing the amount of measurement required. Accurate sampling methods are crucial in supporting any assumption that what you found in your study can be applied back to the larger population that the sample represents. Ideally, your samples are random so that your groups are comparable and your sample adequately reflects the population. Commonly, however, bedside scientists find that random samples are not possible. The examples that follow show a variety of ways to achieve a strong sampling strategy, even with the resource constraints that face most clinicians. As you read the examples, think of ways that you can use simple methods to strengthen your samples and decrease sampling bias.

(continues)

Concepts in Action (continued)

Labor and Delivery Workflow: The Use of Random Selection for Individual Observation

This study was done to understand better what type of care nurses gave to patients in their first stage of labor. Obstetric physicians, nurses, anesthesiologists, nurse practitioners and physician assistants all felt that supportive measures (e.g., positioning and turning patients) could have a significant impact on both mother and baby during the delivery process. In this preintervention and postintervention study, the team hoped to identify what proportion of maternal care was classified as supportive care. If this proportion was low, the team planned to provide education on ways to provide more supportive care.

It was cost and time prohibitive to observe all labor and delivery nurses taking care of patients during their first stage of labor. Thus, instead, the research team chose to randomly select blocks of time and observe randomly selected nurses taking care of one patient in her first stage of labor. To do this, they did some pilot observation to determine how many total observations they needed.

Randomization Method

Because 1 month of shifts was chosen and all shifts needed to be equally represented, all shifts were grouped together. Each shift was numbered. Then random numbers were generated that were between the highest and lowest shift number, and those shifts were selected. Hours of the day were assigned sequential numbers, and random numbers were again generated between 1 and 24.

A different randomization method was chosen for selecting the nurses to observe because each shift would have a different number of nurses caring for mothers in their first stage of labor. When the observer started a shift, he or she identified all nurses taking care of mothers in the first stage of labor and wrote those names on a strip of paper that was folded and put in a container. The container was shaken, and the nurse drew a name. That nurse was observed during the selected time period.

ICU Nurse Workflow: Use of Random Time Assignment for Group Observation

A large 28-bed medical/surgical intensive care unit planned to change many of its processes from manual to electronic. They knew this would have an impact on workflow of all clinicians working in the intensive care

Concepts in Action *(continued)*

unit. They decided to choose one group—nurses—because they were unit based and would likely feel the most impact from the changes in workflow. In order to determine the specific impact of the changes, the study team decided to evaluate workflow before and after the changes were made. It was assumed that the new electronic documentation system would decrease the amount of time that nurses spent charting and increase the amount of time nurses spent in direct patient care (i.e., things such as talking to the patient, doing dressing changes, and turning the patient, that directly impacted the patient's care). To evaluate effectively how this affected the entire unit, the study team decided that they wanted to go beyond observing individual nurses to observing the workflow of the entire unit of nurses.

Observing an entire unit's activities took careful thought and planning. First, the study team developed a task list of all types of nursing tasks and activities. A small group of expert nurse observers was chosen and carefully trained. Agreement between observers was evaluated—that is, that they all identified and categorized the tasks they saw the nurses doing in exactly the same way. A pilot phase of observations was carried out. Based on information from this pilot phase, power and sample sizes were calculated and the number of observations needed was determined. Randomly selected observation times were selected from each of the three shifts: days (0700 to 1459), evenings (1500 to 2259), and nights (2200 to 0659). During those preselected times, the trained nurse observer walked through the entire unit and recorded what task or activity each nurse was doing.

Randomization Method

First, a 2-week block of time was chosen. Then, each day was divided into 15-minute time blocks, as it took a nurse approximately 15 minutes to walk through the two units and observe all of the nurses. Each of these walk-throughs was considered a *round* and was assigned a number. Eighty-four rounds were randomly selected throughout the 2-week period.

Parental Anxiety and Physician Treatment Outcomes: Use of the Entire Population

There was a "gut feel" among pediatricians that a relationship existed between the parent's level of anxiety and their confidence with care of their child. There was concern that this anxiety might impact the way the

(continues)

Concepts in Action *(continued)*

physician chose to treat their child (e.g., order more tests and keep the child in the hospital for extra days).

In this situation, the entire population of all parents of children who were admitted to a pediatric unit with the diagnosis of bronchiolitis was recruited. Non–English-speaking parents or parents who had a history of child abuse were excluded. The bronchiolitis diagnosis was chosen because those parents appeared particularly anxious. The entire population was used because only 20 to 50 patients met the criteria in a year. Often, when populations are small, every potential subject is used because a random selection process would decrease the sample size below a usable level.

Impact of a New Hydrophilic Straight Catheter on Urinary Tract Infections: Use of Convenience Sampling for a Pilot

Hospital-acquired urinary tract infections are often associated with use of a urinary catheter, especially indwelling catheters. To decrease the use of an indwelling catheter in patients who only need intermittent catheterization, a straight catheter is used instead. The process for using the straight catheter was simple: the sterile straight catheter is inserted using sterile technique, the bladder is emptied, and the straight catheter is removed and discarded. This can be uncomfortable to the patient. On one orthopedic unit, straight catheters were used frequently in some patients, and it seemed that a large number of these patients subsequently developed a hospital-acquired urinary tract infection. Working with a quality management team, the unit decided to trial a new straight catheter that was coated with a hydrophilic coating that would make it easier to insert and possibly decrease trauma to the urinary canal.

A *convenience sampling* method was used during the pilot phase. Using this method, all patients admitted to the orthopedic unit during a 1-month period and who had an order for straight catheterization were enrolled in the study. The new hydrophilic straight catheter was used on all patients, and they were evaluated for prevalence of urinary tract infections. Both nurses and patients filled out a questionnaire about their satisfaction with the product. This pilot study gave the team a chance to refine their questionnaire and study methods and provided information that was then used to create a larger study.

Emergency Waiting Room Improvement Study: Using Anonymous Surveys

Many people tend to be less honest and more approving if they know that someone can link their comments to their identity. Understanding

Concepts in Action *(continued)*

this, a team studying emergency department waiting rooms chose to reduce this bias by giving an anonymous survey to patients and their families. The survey itself had few demographics (limited to broad age groupings, gender, and an emergency severity index score) and once the patient or family completed the survey, it was placed in a locked box. Surveys were given to all patients and families who presented to the emergency department during randomly selected time periods. Particularly when sensitive information is gathered or when honesty is a concern, consider methods to retain subject anonymity—such as coding measurement instruments, or omitting any superfluous demographic data—to encourage honest and complete responses.

Comparison of Two Ventilators: Use Inclusion and Exclusion Criteria to Define a Sample

Researchers designed a multisite trial for new-onset adult respiratory distress syndrome patients to compare use of two types of ventilators. Power and sample size calculations made clear that the team would need to select carefully the type of patient entered in the trial. As a result, strict inclusion and exclusion criteria—17 in all—were applied. Because the research focused on unusual cases, this team was actually looking for a sample of outliers. The extensive criteria helped to identify appropriate subjects and narrow the population size. For example, because the primary outcome variable was days on the ventilator from the initial diagnosis of adult respiratory distress syndrome, patients with significant co-morbid conditions were excluded.

Validation of a Pain Tool: A Simple Random Assignment Process

Many measurement tools are developed for acute care and then used in other settings without re-evaluating their population-specific psychometric properties. One long-term care administrator was concerned that the usual pain scale might be misinterpreted by residential patients in long-term care. The administrator decided to conduct reliability testing on the pain scale using residents in the three nursing homes under her management. To select a random sample quickly and easily, the administrator stood in each patient's doorway and flipped a coin. If the coin landed on heads, she invited the resident to participate in the study; if it landed on tails she did not. A random sample was achieved with a minimum of effort.

Secondary Data Collection: A Systematic Sampling Process

A metabolic support team in a Midwestern tertiary-care facility wanted to determine whether early metabolic support (parenteral nutrition) had

(continues)

Concepts in Action *(continued)*

an impact on length of stay in the intensive care unit. The team decided to conduct chart reviews and collect data about the timing of metabolic support consult, days on metabolic support, and length of stay in the intensive care unit. The team conducted a power analysis and determined they needed 85 subjects. After obtaining appropriate permissions, the team narrowed the population to a 6-month period. After reviewing a log of intensive care unit admissions, they calculated a 10% random sample was needed. One member of the team used a table of random numbers to select the starting number, and then every 10th patient was selected from the log.

Checklist for Evaluating the Sampling Plan of a Research Study

_____ The target population is clearly identified.

_____ Inclusion criteria are specific and objective.

_____ Exclusion criteria are specified to control extraneous variables.

_____ Procedures for selecting the sample are specified (if not, assume a convenience sample).

_____ Sampling procedures are likely to produce a representative sample.

_____ Potential for sampling bias has been identified and controlled by the researcher.

_____ The sample is unaffected by common sources of bias such as homogeneity, nonresponse, and systematic attrition.

_____ The sample is of adequate size.

_____ Power analysis is conducted and reported, and is at least 80% (unnecessary if all results were statistically significant).

_____ This sample could reasonably be expected to represent my patients and setting.

CHAPTER 8

Do Not Fear the Numbers

In this chapter, you will learn to

- Focus on the most important numbers in the results section of a research report
- Determine the effect of power on a study
- Decide whether reliability and validity are acceptable for the measures used
- Evaluate hypothesis tests for appropriateness and significance
- Strengthen the statistical analysis of your practice-based studies

You are reading an excellent article on the effects of a collaborative patient education plan on patient compliance. The authors conclude that patient education plans that are interdisciplinary lead to better compliance on the part of the patient. Primary care physicians, nurses, therapists, nutritionists, and pharmacists worked on an integrated teaching plan; the authors claim that they can explain nearly 50% of patient compliance efforts by the amount of interdisciplinary patient education that is provided. You wonder how that is possible—to predict patient behaviors. It seems exciting and makes you think of several research questions that you could answer with this technique. The methods, procedures, and measures all seem pretty straightforward. Then you get to the analysis—tables follow tables with numbers that mean nothing to you; the text is full of references to power, p values, beta coefficients, test statistics, and r-

139

squared—this seems like a foreign language to you. After trying to wade through the results, you are not sure which numbers are important and which are not. Apparently, the authors were able to predict the overall outcome as well as the effect of each clinician's relative contribution. After trying to follow the text and decipher the tables, you finally give up and jump to the discussion section. Ah! Back to words! This part makes sense. You wish you could decide for yourself whether you believe the author's conclusions—but you cannot even tell which numbers are important, let alone whether the authors used them correctly. "I will just have to trust them," you think to yourself, "and hope they know what they are doing."

The statistical analysis of a research study provides the tools to determine whether interventions do, indeed, make a difference. Without statistical analysis, a researcher cannot quantify whether results are attributable to the experiment or to some random effect. Yet the statistical section of a research article is often a mystery to the practicing clinician, a collection of tables, figures, and numbers that sometimes confuses more than they clarify. For most clinicians, statistics courses are a remote memory. Thus, the results section of a research article—thick with a daunting array of numbers, symbols, and unfamiliar abbreviations—is often passed over. It is common for clinicians to focus on the methods and then flip to the discussion section, taking on faith that the statistics were appropriate.

The results section, however, is simply a collection of numbers, and numbers are just tools—tools that are used to convert results into information. Numbers are used in research to measure the effects of sampling, quantify the amount of error in measurement, and put a value on the effects of chance. The numbers in a research study can help us decide whether the findings are clinically relevant and whether the effect of a treatment is big enough to be of practical use. Numbers give us a yardstick to assess whether estimates are precise and useful. Ultimately, the numbers in a research study help us decide whether the results are credible and whether we should apply the findings to our own practice.

That is not to say that the bedside scientist must understand every statistical test and interpret each numerical result to determine whether results are credible. Understanding the ways numbers are used, combined with a focus on some specific numbers that are important in any research study, can help us determine whether the results can be trusted.

Not all important numbers are located in the statistical results section of a research study. There are numbers throughout a study—from the descriptors of the sample to the psychometric properties of instruments to the actual test statistics—that help us assess the credibility of a study. A general understanding of these numbers is sufficient to judge the usefulness of a study for practice.

The most important numbers in a study are those that describe the sample, quantify the amount of error in the measurements, calculate the magnitude of the effect (if there is one), calculate the probability that chance was responsible for the outcome, and assess the amount of uncertainty in estimates. Each has some straightforward rules for appropriate use and interpretation.

NUMBERS THAT DESCRIBE THE SAMPLE

Several numbers in a research study describe the sample. Quantification of characteristics of the sample is important for many reasons. Numbers relative to the sample can tell us whether the experimental and control groups are similar enough to control extraneous variables. Information about the size of samples and the way sample size was determined is particularly important in deciding whether the results of statistical tests can be trusted.

Numbers that Describe Group Comparability

Deciding whether results are due to a treatment requires that other explanations for a result are eliminated. Differences in key characteristics of subjects—such as age, severity of illness, co-morbid conditions, or ethnicity for example—may compromise internal validity. The effects of these extraneous variables can be minimized if they are distributed equally between the experimental and control groups.

Some researchers use matching to assure that subjects are similar in both groups. Matching means that subjects with characteristics that might affect the experiment are placed into the experimental and the control group in the same proportion. Matching is a strong method for assuring groups are similar, but this strategy is not always possible. In these cases, the researcher can achieve nearly the same end by statistically determining if groups are equal after the fact. Testing for differences between groups on key characteristics strengthens a study. If groups are statistically equal on key characteristics (particularly those that might be extraneous variables), then randomization has been successful in distributing these characteristics equally across all groups. When groups have been evaluated for comparability, the researcher should provide the results of inferential tests to determine whether the groups are the same on key characteristics. In this case, the statistical tests should be *not* significant—meaning that any differences between groups are due to chance. When tests of group comparability are provided in a research study, look for a p value that is *greater than 0.05*, meaning that the groups are statistically identical.

Numbers that Describe Power

The size of a sample should be determined objectively, based on the process of power analysis. Described in detail in Chapter 7, power is the capacity of a sample to detect a difference between groups if a difference does indeed exist. Sufficient power controls type II error and builds confidence in the study findings (particularly if they were *not* statistically significant). Power should be calculated and reported by the authors, either prospectively or retrospectively. A power of at least 80% is the minimum acceptable level.

Calculations of power are based on the expected variability in the sample, the amount of difference that would be considered important, and the amount of error that is considered tolerable by the authors. A researcher should provide the reader with these numerical assumptions and describe the method by which power was calculated.

Sometimes, prospective power calculation is impossible, and retrospective power is calculated. Retrospective power calculation involves calculating the amount of power a sample actually possessed, after data have already been collected. Either method is acceptable, as sufficient power is documented by either prospective or retrospective methods. Prospective power calculation does have the advantage of assuring sufficient subjects will be included up front so that a lack of power is not an expected reason for insignificant findings. Retrospective power analysis has the disadvantage of documenting insufficient power after data collection is complete, when increasing sample size may be difficult, untimely, or impossible.

Authors may not report power if results are significant. Because insufficient power is only an issue if no significant results are found, if results are significant, the study clearly had sufficient power. Look for numbers reflecting power in the section of a research study that describes the sample. A researcher may report beta, which is the risk of a type II error. Power is calculated as 1-beta, and thus, a beta of 0.15 means 1 minus 0.15 or 85% power. Look for a number documented as either a decimal (at least 0.85) or a percentage (85%). Power is a direct function of sample size; larger samples in general have more power, and a researcher can increase power by increasing the number of subjects.

Numbers that Describe Sample Size

Power is affected by sample size, but the number of subjects in an experiment affects virtually all aspects of the statistical analysis. The size of the sample constrains the number and type of tests that can be run on the data. If multiple tests are run, then larger samples are needed. Sample size also re-

From the Mouths of Bedside Scientists: How Clinicians Talk About Statistics

Why is it important for clinicians to understand statistics?

I have been a practicing nurse for 32 years. Today, there is a need to provide safe, quality care using cost-effective methods. To do that, clinicians need to be able to understand the reasoning behind necessary changes in practice. We can no longer afford "sacred cow" thinking to guide our actions. We have to seek out and understand research studies—and their statistical analysis—in order to evaluate and change practice. These changes should happen, however, only if there truly is good reasoning and data to substantiate the change.

How can clinicians use statistics?

Statistics can help clinicians to assess diagnoses and treatments better. Much of medical treatment deals with what has and has not worked with past patients. Using statistical data, one can figure out how different medicines or treatments work with the *average* patient. In addition, documenting progress with data is a statistical function that we use all of the time.

What does a p value mean to you?

A p value determines whether the results are simply due to chance or whether they are a true test result. Small p values indicate the results were very unlikely due to chance. In this case, confidence levels would be high that the treatment has produced real results.

What do you look for in the statistical section before you will use a study in your practice?

Before understanding the basic principles of statistics, I read any type of article from a professional journal and thought it was valid, simply because it was printed in a respected journal. Now that I have a greater understanding of statistical analysis and the "how" and "why" of different tests, I can tell when there is a discrepancy between what the actual statistical results are and the conclusions that have been drawn by the authors. Now I take more caution when reading research in journals and am careful only to use research that has high credibility from valid statistical processes.

stricts the number of comparisons that can be made between variables or subgroups, such as gender. When the researcher has run multiple tests, compared many subgroups, and has a lot of variables in the analysis, the sample size should get larger.

The size of a sample lets the researcher assume whether to expect a normal distribution of data, as well. A normal distribution—or data that fall into a bell curve—is an assumption for most inferential statistical tests. Calculation of the p value (probability of chance) and the selection of a specific hypothesis test are both based on whether the data are normally distributed. When small samples are used—in general, less than 30—then a normal distribution cannot be assumed. Small samples may have distributions that are skewed, meaning that the data are higher at one end or the other of the distribution. When samples are smaller than 200, the author should test for normal distribution and report the results, and thus, the reader can be assured the right tests have been applied.

How big of a sample is adequate? Calculating power ensures adequacy of sample size, but if power calculation is not reported, some general rules can be used to do a basic evaluation of sample size adequacy:

- In general, 30 subjects in each group give you greater confidence that a normal distribution was achieved. It may be questionable to generalize results from studies with fewer than 30 subjects, particularly if the author is concluding the treatment has no effect.
- Although a great deal of controversy exists about the number of subjects needed for multiple comparisons, the rule is that 15 subjects should be included for every variable studied. This number increases when subgroups are compared.
- When subjects are studied with surveys, regardless of the ultimate size of the sample, a *response* rate of at least 50% is needed to draw valid conclusions.
- Samples will need to be larger when there is a great deal of variability in a sample, as heterogeneous samples have greater sampling error. Variability is evaluated with the standard deviation. As a stand-alone statistic, the standard deviation is not very meaningful, but if compared with the mean value, it can reflect heterogeneity of the sample. A large standard deviation *relative to the mean* indicates a large amount of variability in the sample, and more subjects will be needed to achieve adequate power.

Although a small sample does not universally compromise the validity of the study, the results should be assessed with the caution that type II error may be an explanation for insignificant results. When conducting a systematic review, sample size issues become less of a concern when multiple studies reflect the same findings.

Where to Look for Information About Statistical Results

The statistical results of a study are easy to identify. Most often labeled "results," the numbers generally appear in tables and graphs as well as imbedded in the text. It is a commonly accepted format to report the results without any interpretive comment and then to follow with a discussion of what the numbers mean. Thus, it is not a weakness if the statistical section reads like a numerical report, without comment about the importance of the numbers.

Inspect the tables carefully, and assure that they match the way the results are reported in textual form. The numerical tables should include *at least* the tests that were run, the associated test statistics, and a p value for each test. Sometimes, the p values are reported with an asterisk (*) or some other identifier, with a subscript to the table identifying the codes for p values as less than 0.05, 0.01, and 0.001. A lack of an identifier usually means that the result was not statistically significant. P values are not reported as "0.000," even if that was the calculated value, as a researcher will generally not conclude that there was absolutely no effect of sampling error. In these cases, the p value is usually reported as "< 0.001," indicating that the effects of chance were not measurable.

If a statistic is followed by a range of numbers in parentheses, the author has included confidence intervals. This strengthens the study, as confidence intervals help you to evaluate both the precision of the estimate and how close the results were to significance. The confidence interval may be reported as a simple range of numbers (7.6 to 9.8) or as a number with a $\pm$ range after it (7.0 $\pm$ 1.5.) The latter indicates that the confidence interval is 5.5 (7.0 $-$ 1.5) to 8.5 (7.0 $+$ 1.5.) Either is an acceptable way to report confidence intervals.

Not all of the important numbers are located in the results section. Look for numbers that describe group comparability and power in the section that describes the sampling strategy. If there is no separate section for the sampling procedure, then tests of group comparability and power analysis should be the first numbers reported in the results section. The authors may report power as a percentage (80%) or a decimal number (0.80) or even a whole number (80). Alternatively, some authors report beta (b). Power is 1-beta, and thus, subtracting the reported beta from 1 will give the sample power. In other words, if an author reports a beta of 0.15, the power is 85%.

Reliability statistics are most commonly reported in the methods and procedures section, when measurements and instrumentation are described. Ideally, the authors will report both the types of reliability and validity that were tested and the resulting statistics. The best reports include reliability testing from the instrument's developers as well as from the current sample.

Numbers That Describe Sampling Error

If a researcher could include every member of a population in his or her study, then sampling error would be nonexistent. That is rarely possible, however; thus, it is inevitable that there will be some differences between the characteristics of a population and the characteristics of the sample, no matter how carefully the sample is drawn. These differences are quantified as standard error and are directly affected by variability and indirectly affected by sample size. As samples get larger, standard error gets smaller.

How big is a standard error that is unacceptable? There is no easy answer for that question—standard error is a relative number, specific to the measures that are used and their scale. However, when a standard error is very large relative to the mean value, you can draw the conclusion that a lot of sampling error is present in the experiment. Because standard error is, in general, the comparison value to determine statistical significance, it may be difficult to find statistically significant results when standard error is large. The researcher can reduce standard error by using a sound sampling strategy and drawing a sample that is as large as is practical.

The size of the sample and the error associated with sampling both contribute to the power of an experiment. You should assess numbers that reflect this error—calculation of power, sample size, and standard error—to determine whether the sample is sufficient for the conclusions drawn. Even when sampling error is small and the sample size is large, however, misleading results may be caused by error associated with the measurement itself. Measurement error can be directly evaluated if the authors provide numbers that reflect the reliability and validity of the measures that are used.

NUMBERS THAT DESCRIBE THE MEASUREMENTS

Measurement is a key element in research. As described in Chapter 6, the measures can consistently report accurate values, or they can be unreliable and create threats to validity. The amount of error in the measurement can be quantified and should be reported, and thus, the reader can decide whether measurement error impacts the outcome of the study.

Numbers that Describe Reliability of the Measures

Reliability of measurement was described in depth in Chapter 6. Reliability reflects consistency and determines the amount of precision that is achieved with the measures. Measures of internal reliability (coefficient alpha, Cronbach's alpha) should exceed 0.7. Measures of split-half reliability should exceed 0.6; measures of test–retest reliability and parallel reliability should exceed 0.5.

If the author provides statistical evidence of reliability, it allows for more than a general assessment of precision. Measurement error can be directly calculated from a reliability coefficient. Subtracting the internal reliability coefficient from 1.0 quantifies the amount of error in the measure. For example, if the reported coefficient alpha is 0.93, then the measurement contributes $1 - 0.93$ or 7% measurement error to the experiment.

What is measurement error? Measurement error is defined as the difference between the *measured* or *observed* score and the *true score*. A low level of measurement error supports internal validity because differences that are detected between groups can be attributed to real differences and not to differences in the actual measures. When sampling error and measurement error are both minimized, then differences between groups can be reasonably attributed to the treatment effect and not to the effects of sampling or measurement.

NUMBERS THAT DESCRIBE THE EFFECTS OF TREATMENTS

In general, the point of inferential statistics is to tell us whether groups are truly different from each other on some outcome or dependent variable. Although inferential statistics often *are* complicated, there are really only three reported statistics that you must be able to interpret to tell if a study should be applied to your patients: (1) the p value, which tells us whether the differences are *real*; (2) the test statistic, which tells us if the differences are *important*; and (3) confidence intervals, which tell us how *precise* the estimates are. All three of these statistics should be taken together to determine the significance of the findings for practice.

The P Value: Is the Difference Real?

Much has been made of the p value and statistical significance in research. In fact, many novice researchers focus on little else. Yet statistical significance gives us only this information about research results: a small p value indicates that findings are not due to sampling error. This is important to know—it helps us to evaluate whether differences between groups are due to sampling error or are attributable to the treatment. The p value, however, does not tell us whether the findings are important, or of practical use, or applicable to our patients. Thus, we start by looking at the p value but only because if results are not statistically significant, there is not much point in looking any further. If the only differences are those that are due to sampling error, then practical applications are irrelevant.

Hitting the Stacks

Kuppermann et al. (2004) studied the effect of hysterectomy versus medical treatment on quality of life and sexual function. This was a multicenter, randomized controlled trial in which the independent variable was treatment for abnormal uterine bleeding; the primary outcome measures were physical health, symptom resolution, body image, and sexual function. Statistics were reported for all the major aspects of the study. "A sample size of at least 60 participants would allow us to reject the null hypothesis of no difference . . . with 90% power in a two-sided test with an alpha of 0.05. . . . We observed a nominally significant difference among 20 comparisons of the baseline characteristics of the randomized groups [p = .11 to .93] indicating the randomization was technically successful. . . . At 6 months, women in the hysterectomy group had greater improvement in symptom resolution (75 vs. 29, p < .001), symptom satisfaction (44 vs. 7, p < .001), interference with sex (41 vs. 22, p = .003), sexual desire (21 vs. 3, p = .01), health distress (33 vs. 13, p = .009), sleep problems (13 vs. 1, p = .03), overall health (12 vs. 2, p = .006), and satisfaction with health (31 vs. 14, p = .01.)"

Aly et al. (2004) studied the effects of physical activity combined with massage on bone mineralization in premature infants. This randomized trial involved 30 preterm infants assigned to either a treatment group (a daily protocol of massage and physical activity) or a control group that received neither of these measures. Biomarkers of bone formation and resorption (serum calcium, alkaline phosphatase, procollagen type I C-terminal propeptide [PICP]) were measured at study entry and at 1.8 kg of body weight. "We hypothesized that our intervention would increase the group difference in PICP by threefold. When we used the baseline value from a previous study and assumed a correlation coefficient (r = .7) between pre- and post intervention observations, a sample of 30 subjects (15 in each group) would detect that difference with power = .80 . . . and alpha = 0.05 level of significance. . . . The groups were similar in gestational age, birth weight, and gender distribution. They also had no significant differences in caloric, calcium, or protein intake over the study period [p = .081 to .984]. . . . Both groups had an increase in serum calcium levels over the course of the study. The relative percent increase was higher in the activity group (19.5%) than in the control group (4.3%) p = 0.002."

Kuppermann, M., R. Varner, R. Summitt, L. Learman, C. Ireland, E. Vittinghoff, A. Stewart, F. Lin, H. Richter, J. Showstack, S. Hulley, and A. Washington. 2004. Effect of hysterectomy vs. medical treatment on health-related quality of life and sexual functioning. *Journal of the American Medical Association* 291: 1447–55.

Aly, H., M. Moustafa, S. Hassanein, A. Massaro, H. Amer, and K. Patel. 2004. Physical activity combined with massage improves bone mineralization in premature infants: A randomized trial. *Journal of Perinatology* 24: 305–9.

With that being said, the p value is an easy statistic to interpret. It is interpreted virtually the same in every experiment, regardless of the tests used. Focus for a bit on what the p value represents: it is the probability that results are due to error. Thus, it makes sense that we would want the probability of error to be very small. Two comparison levels are used for the p value in most biomedical experiments—0.05 and on occasion 0.01. The lower the p value, the more confident we can be that the differences are not due to sampling error.

The researcher should tell the reader up front what level of comparison has been set for the study. This level of comparison is referred to as alpha and represents the amount of error the researcher is willing to tolerate. This is called type I error. Type I error is considered the most serious error in biomedical experiments, as it is essentially concluding that a treatment makes a difference when it does not. (This alpha is a different number than Cronbach's alpha or the alpha reliability coefficient. The reliability alpha is a calculated statistic; this alpha is a preset standard for statistical significance.) Thus, if alpha is set at 0.05, then the researcher is willing to tolerate a 5% probability that results may be due to sampling error. If alpha is set at 0.01, then the researcher can only tolerate 1% risk of error. Five percent is by far more common and is considered the default alpha for most experiments.

If alpha represents tolerable error, why would we not want the lowest possible value for every experiment? When alpha is set very low—say 1%—then we have a very low potential for saying a treatment works when it does not. In other words, 99% of the time, when we say a treatment works, it really does.

If alpha is set very low, however, then the risk increases that there will be a meaningful difference between groups, and we will not find it. For example, if we set alpha at 1%, there can be a 2% chance the results are due to sampling error, and we will not identify it. When a difference exists but we say it does not, we have type II error. Type II error is represented by beta. Setting alpha at a very low level has a tradeoff—an increase in type II error. Setting alpha is based on a consideration of the risks of both type I and type II errors.

In general, the p value should be very low. P values below 5% are often referred to as *statistically significant*, meaning that they are not due to sampling error. The actual p value may be reported (e.g., $p = 0.036$) or numerical results may have a notation, with a subscript to the table indicating that noted statistics are statistically significant at 0.05. P values as small as 0.01, 0.001, or 0.005 are often reported, indicating a high degree of statistical significance. When the p value has been calculated as 0.000, then it is usually reported as < 0.001 because few researchers will go so far as to say there is *no* risk of error.

Look for a Small P Value Associated with Each Test

If the p value is larger than 0.05, then the results may well be due to sampling error and are not statistically significant. If the p value is smaller than 0.05—regardless of how it is reported—then the findings are *real* and not due to error or chance. This is the first step in determining whether findings should be applied to other situations. On the other hand, in order to determine whether findings are important, then we need to look directly at the test statistic.

NUMBERS THAT REPORT THE TEST STATISTIC

A test statistic is a ratio that compares differences in the data to those that would occur purely by chance because of sampling error. The larger this ratio gets, the greater the difference between the results and error. The choice of a test statistic is determined by many aspects of a research study:

- The research question may dictate a particular analytic test.
- The level of measurement may constrain the choice of tests.
- The distribution of the variable values may restrict the tests that can be run.
- The sample size may limit the tests that can be used.
- The expected relationship between variables may require a particular statistic.

The Research Question

Some research questions dictate specific methods of analysis. If the words *relationship* or *association* appear in the research question, then correlation or chi-square statistics should be used. If the words *differences* or *cause and effect* are implied by the research question, then inferential tests of group differences are required, such as t tests, analysis of variance, or Mann-Whitney U. If *explanation* or *prediction* occurs in the research question, then regression tests should be used. The research question will also drive the choice of variables and the level at which they are measured.

The Level of Measurement

Not all numbers are created the same, and not all numbers in a research study can be treated the same way mathematically. *Nominal* data are those that can be placed into categories, but cannot be ranked. Nominal data include, for example, gender, marital status, ethnicity, diagnosis, and other variables that can be named but not measured on a scale. Nominal data can be counted, and thus, frequencies, percentages, proportions, and rates can all be determined from nominal values. When nominal data can fall into only two categories (e.g., gender or mortality), then they are often referred to as binomial or dichotomous.

Strengthen Your Statistical Analysis

Not everyone is a statistical expert—or needs to be. Statistics is a highly specialized area of applied mathematics that takes time and education to master. However, there are still measures you can take to assure that your research conclusions are statistically sound and reported accurately:

- Approach your analysis systematically, focusing on the four most important areas of statistical reporting: sample power, measurement reliability, tests of group equivalency, and tests of treatment effects. Describe each area in words, and make decisions about such things as acceptable error, expected power, and precision before thinking about which tests to use.

- Consult someone who is good with statistics before collecting data. An individual with statistical expertise may not necessarily be a statistician; the quality department, infection control, medical staff, and marketing may all have people who are good with statistical analysis. Talk over your design early, as it is too late to modify your analysis after data are already collected.

- Create a dummy data collection sheet before you collect any data. You will often find the weaknesses of your data analysis plan when you try to set up the analysis of the data. Walk through the data collection and analysis with a dummy spreadsheet before your data collection plan is complete, and modify your plan to avoid difficulties later.

- Hindsight is 20/20, and you will find the weaknesses of your data when you try to conduct analyses. Do not be discouraged; do find someone with statistical expertise to help you sort through what you can and cannot do with the numbers.

Ordinal data are categorical data that can be put in rank order. A pain scale is an example of ordinal data. Patients are asked to place themselves in one of the categories represented by the scale, denoting a relative value from a great deal of pain to very little pain. There is a high and low end of the scale—or bad and good, big and little—so that the categories can be ranked. This ranking gives the researcher a bit more versatility in the statistics that can be used in analysis. These data can still be counted and expressed in any way a frequency can be expressed, but in addition, the minimum, maximum, and median data can also be identified and tested. The primary distinction of ordinal

Table 8-1   Appropriate Summary Statistics by Level of Measurement

Level of Measurement	Distributions	Averages	Dispersion	Shape
Nominal	Frequency Percentage	Mode		
Ordinal	Frequency Percentage	Mode Median	Range Minimum/ Maximum	
Interval/Ratio		Mode Median Mean	Range Minimum/Maximum Standard Deviation Variance	Skew Kurtosis

data is that the entries on the scale cannot be directly compared *across* the scale, because we do not know that the intervals between entries are the same. For example, is the difference between "strongly agree" and "agree" exactly the same amount of agreement as the difference between "disagree" and "neutral?" Is the difference between 7 and 8 on the Beck Depression Scale the exact same amount of depression in an older patient and a postpartum mom? Is an independent chair-to-bed transfer Functional Independence Measure (FIM) score the same for a paraplegic and a stroke victim? Although these measures are important, we do not necessarily know that each score or interval is comparable. Thus, we cannot treat the intervals between entries as equal and concurrently lose the ability to do mathematical operations, such as division. This limits what we can do with ordinal data to testing their relative value, frequency, or ranking. Table 8-1 identifies appropriate summary methods for each level of measurement.

Together, nominal and ordinal data are sometimes referred to as categorical, or classification data. Group differences on nominal and ordinal data are tested with a group of tests described as nonparametric, meaning that the tests do not require a normal distribution (bell curve). Some common nonparametric tests are the chi-square tests (goodness of fit, independence, association), the Mann-Whitney U (a test of the median), and the Wilcoxon rank sum (a test of rankings).

For more depth and detail, try these resources:

DeMets, D. 2005. Statistical issues in interpreting clinical trials. *Journal of Internal Medicine Supplement* 742, 257: 56–65.

Fields, A. 2000. *Discovering Statistics Using SPSS for Windows: Advanced Techniques for the Beginner.* London: Sage.

Kranzler, J. 2003. *Statistics for the Terrified,* 3rd ed. Upper Saddle River, NJ: Prentice-Hall.

Machin, D. 2005. On the evolution of statistical methods as applied to clinical trials. *Journal of Internal Medicine Supplement* 742, 257: 48–54.

Mason, M. 1999. A review of procedural and statistical methods for handling attrition and missing data in clinical research. *Measurement and Evaluation in Counseling and Development.* 32: 111–9.

Newton, R., and K. Rudestam. 1999. *Your Statistical Consultant.* Thousand Oaks, CA: Sage.

Norman, G., and D. Streiner. 2003. *PDQ (Pretty Darned Quick) Statistics,* 3rd ed. Hamilton, Ontario: BC Decker.

Parker, R., and D. Brossart. 2003. Evaluating single case research data: A comparison of seven statistical methods. *Behavior Therapy* 34: 189–212.

Porschan, M. 1999. Statistical methods for monitoring clinical trials. *Journal of Biopharmaceutical Statistics* 9: 599–616.

Wang, S., H. Hung, and Y. Tsong. 2002. Utility and pitfalls of some statistical methods in active controlled clinical trials. *Controlled Clinical Trials* 23: 15–29.

Nominal and ordinal data are attractive because they are simple to collect. Subjects are placed in categories or some response is placed in rank order. The attractiveness of their simplicity is balanced by the relative insensitivity of the measures and the limitations of data that are not normally distributed. There are relatively few tests that run well on nonnormally distributed data, and they are not very sensitive; thus, large samples are needed.

When sample sizes exceed about 200, however, the limitations of ordinal data are of less concern. Large samples—no matter what the level of measurement—tend to take on a normal distribution. We do not have this concern at all when using interval or ratio level data, as we can make more assumptions about these numbers.

Interval data are data that are measured on a scale. The scale theoretically has an infinite number of entries, and a subject can fall anywhere on the scale (not just in categories.) The size of intervals between measurement units is identical, no matter where it falls on the scale. For example, a centimeter will always be a centimeter, no matter whether it falls between 10 and 11 centimeters or between 150 and 151. The intervals between entries are also proportionate, meaning that 20 units are twice as big as 10, which is twice as big as five. This equality of intervals gives us more confidence that the data will be normally distributed—in a bell curve—and that mathematical operations are trustworthy.

When interval data have a true zero, then they are considered a ratio scale. This distinction is not of major importance in interpreting statistics, however, unless the tests are extraordinarily sensitive or the sample extremely small. Interval and ratio data together are often referred to as continuous data. They are considered discrete if the units can only be measured in whole numbers, such as number of children, or illnesses requiring surgery.

A wide range of inferential tests is available for interval and ratio data. Analysis of variance, t tests, and linear regression are some of the more common tests used on these data.

After the research question has been specified and the variables defined, the level of measurement of each can be evaluated and an appropriate group of tests identified. The selection of a specific test depends on the specific statistic from the data that will be tested.

The Selection of a Specific Test

The final selection of a specific test depends on the statistics that are used to represent the variables. For example, when testing interval level data, means are often used to represent a typical response. Tests of means include several varieties of the t test or analysis of variance. Frequencies, proportions, and rates are tested with chi-square.

The choice should also take into consideration the relationship that is expected between variables. Association and relationship are tested with different statistics than are the effects of treatments. Sample size will also support or limit the selection of a specific test. Table 8-2 reviews some of the most common statistics used in research.

When these tests are reported, two numbers should be included: the actual test statistic and its associated p value. The relative size of the test statistic can indicate *magnitude of effect* or the size of the differences between groups. This allows you to conclude whether the difference is large enough to be of practical use. For example, if a nutritionist were studying whether a

Table 8-2   Some Common Statistics, Their Use, and Interpretation

Statistical Test	What It Is Used For	It May Be Called . . .	Symbols	Interpretation
Chi-square	Used to analyze nominal, ordinal, or binomial data, expressed as percentages, frequencies, proportions, or rates Common tests are test of independence of two samples; test of goodness of fit of a single sample and a known population value; test of an association between two variables in a single sample	Pearson chi-square Fisher's exact test Likelihood ratio Cross-tabs Mantel-Haenszel	χ^2	A large chi-square value usually indicates a difference in values or an association between variables; check that associated p values are less than 0.05 to confirm statistical significance
T test	Used to analyze interval or ratio level data expressed as mean scores, between two groups. (When more than two groups are analyzed, analysis of variance is more appropriate.) Common tests are one-sample tests between a sample mean	Student's t test	t	A large t value usually indicates a significant difference, but significance depends on sample size as well; check that associated p values are less than 0.05 to confirm statistical significance

(continues)

Table 8-2   Some Common Statistics, Their Use, and Interpretation *(continued)*

Statistical Test	What It Is Used For	It May Be Called . . .	Symbols	Interpretation
	and a known population mean; independent samples tests between two samples; paired sample tests between two related samples			
Alpha	Preset standard for statistical significance; represents the risk of error the researcher is willing to accept	Significance level	α	Usually set at 0.05 If set at a different level (a common alternative is 0.01) the researcher should provide a rationale for the choice
Alpha coefficient	Test of the internal reliability of a measurement instrument	Cronbach's alpha Internal alpha Internal reliability	α	> 0.7 is desirable; > 0.9 is strong
Correlation coefficient	Descriptive measure of the strength and direction of a relationship between two variables in a sample	Pearson's product moment correlation Spearman's rank	ρ, r, or rho	A negative sign indicates an inverse relationship; a positive sign indicates a positive relationship; > 0.7 indicates a relationship, > 0.9 a strong one

nutritional supplement was helpful in supporting weight gain in cancer patients, a difference in weight of 4 ounces might be statistically significant if the sampling error is low. If the difference is applied to a preterm neonate, this might be of great practical use. However, what if the patients are 50-year-old men? Would a weight gain of one-fourth pound be of practical use? This small of an effect might be *real*, but not necessarily *important*. The magnitude of effect helps you make the critical decision of whether to use the results with your patients.

How do you know when a test statistic is large? Again, this is a relative number. In general, the larger the test statistic, the greater the difference detected. Test statistics that are decimals or low single digits may have very little practical effect, even if the p value shows statistical significance. Test statistics that are in the tens or hundreds usually indicate a good deal of effect. When test statistics show a great deal of effect, then the final consideration is how much confidence you have that this statistic can estimate the effect on another population with accuracy.

NUMBERS THAT REFLECT CONFIDENCE IN ESTIMATES

When a test statistic is reported, the researcher may report confidence intervals for the results. Confidence intervals indicate the precision with which the researcher has been able to estimate various characteristics or differences between groups. Confidence intervals get larger as they get less precise; they get smaller as they get more accurate.

Several characteristics of the data can affect the precision of confidence intervals. Large samples, in general, will have more precise estimates. When samples have a lot of variability, on the other hand, there is less precision in estimates. How much confidence is needed affects the size of the interval. For example, if you must be 99% sure that an estimate actually contains the value, then you will need a wider interval to capture it. If 95% is good enough, the interval can get smaller.

Looking at a confidence interval with the test statistic can give you an idea whether the results were "close" or whether the results are precise enough for generalization. For example, if the confidence interval for a mean difference is 0.01 to 6.5, the average difference could be as little as 1/100 unit or as big as 6.5 units. In other words, the difference *could be* next to nothing. On the other hand, if a confidence interval for a mean difference indicated 12.6 to 12.8, not only can we tell that there were quite a few units of average difference between groups, but the estimation of the difference is very precise.

Another Way to Look at It

Confidence intervals tell us how *close our estimates are* to reality. A confidence interval lets us evaluate whether our estimates are precise and to assess whether we are comfortable accepting the researcher's conclusions. Thus, it makes sense that we want the most accurate and precise estimates possible. There are many aspects of data that can affect the precision of estimates. Some of these include sample size, confidence level, and variability.

My niece Steffi is a hotshot basketball player. In her early teens, she won eighth in a national hoops competition, shooting 24 out of 25 free throws in a scenario that would stress out a yoga teacher. She is naturally gifted, athletically built, and her skill has been nurtured since she was a toddler. It is her hard work, however, that has gotten her the kudos she deserves.

I have tremendous confidence in Steffi's ability to hit the basket when she shoots. Part of my confidence comes from knowing the truly enormous number of baskets that she has shot in her young life. Over and over, day after day, she devotes substantial time and effort to practice. Her sample size of baskets is huge. I, on the other hand, shoot baskets once or twice a decade. So whose precision in shooting baskets would you have more confidence in—my ability to hit the basket based on a sample size of a couple dozen or Steffi's with a sample size of several thousand? I am putting my money on the kid.

We do not have so much luck when we go to the county fair, however. Although it should be a walk in the park, Steffi does not hit the baskets so well when she is trying for the large stuffed panda. Why? Because those baskets are smaller than usual—about an inch smaller all around—thus, they are harder to hit. I cannot have as much confidence when the interval that has to be hit is small. If I need a great deal of confidence, then I need a bigger basket.

Part of Steffi's skill is rooted in talent, part in practice, and part in the consistency that comes from a focus on form. When Steffi shoots, each time, she goes through the same rituals, the same motions, the same muscle moves. This lack of variability leads to bigger confidence in her ability to get the job done, and done exactly right.

Confidence in our estimates and their precision then is about more than math. It is about having samples that are big enough to be able to focus our estimates more precisely. It is about setting your confidence estimate at the right level for the precision that you will need, and it is about minimizing variability so that a consistent, accurate answer can be derived. All of these measures can make our estimates more precise and, as a result, more useful.

SUMMARY

All of these numbers taken together help us to determine how much confidence *we* have in the results of a study. Power lets us know whether we could reasonably expect that differences in groups were detected. Sample size also drives the number of variables that can be measured and the volume of tests that can be run. Variability in the sample and sample size together make up sampling error. Reliability coefficients can help us directly quantify measurement error.

Differences between groups are evaluated with the p value, test statistic, and confidence intervals. The p value indicates the probability that results are due to chance, and thus, very small p values indicate a difference is *real*. The test statistic reflects how big the differences are, or the magnitude of effect. Confidence intervals give us information about the precision of estimates. A focus on these numbers in a results section helps simplify interpretation and demystify the analysis of research data.

Concepts in Action

Data collection issues can make or break your study. The following examples describe some innovative ways that investigators deal with the challenge of collecting data efficiently and accurately. As you read these examples, think about your data collection needs, and map out potential issues related to your data collection methods. These examples demonstrate that a bedside science project does not require complicated or lengthy data collection processes; indeed, sometimes the simplest procedures encourage the best completion rates. Thinking about these potential issues early in the research process can help you find alternatives and overcome obstacles so that your conclusions are based on solid data sets.

Music and Anxiety: Use of a Visual Analog Scale

This study compared the use of music to antianxiety medication in relieving mild anxiety in psychiatric inpatients. Antianxiety medication can have side effects such as lethargy, dependency, and decreased alertness. Music can have a calming effect without any associated side effects and can be used without a physician's prescription. These researchers wanted to see whether music worked as well as medication in treating anxiety.

Data were collected directly from the subjects. Patients in the study were given two reliable and valid 20-question anxiety questionnaires. The intent

(continues)

Concepts in Action (continued)

of one questionnaire was to evaluate whether the subject was an anxious person in general, and the other instrument evaluated their current level of anxiety. Both questionnaires were administered on enrollment in the study, and then again on day 3. A visual analog scale (VAS) was shown to the patient when they reported they were feeling anxious. This VAS was a 100-mm visual scale with the words "no anxiety" and "worst possible anxiety" written on the ends (Figure 8-1). The subjects were asked to place a check mark on a line to indicate their level of anxiety. The VAS response was recorded again after they used either antianxiety medication or music to calm their anxiety. The type of medication the patient was using (e.g., benzodiazepine), the dose of medication, and the medication frequency were recorded for all patients enrolled in the study. Although the initial instruments took several minutes for the subjects to complete, the VAS was quick and easy to use for data collection.

Data Collection Challenges
During a pilot phase of 10 patients, the study team discovered that nurses were often rating the VAS themselves and would even write in the approximate percentage by their "X." Additional education was given to staff on the correct way to rate the VAS, using the patient's response. Also, many of the anxiety questionnaires from the pilot could not be found, and thus, for the actual study, a system was developed so that nurses could place the questionnaires in a convenient, locked file after the patient completed the questionnaire.

Physician–Patient Communication Study: Using a Simple Label for Daily Collection

Do physicians communicate with their medical intensive care unit (ICU) patients on a daily basis? Are patients satisfied with their physician's daily communication? Satisfaction with physician communication is part

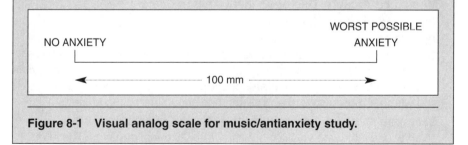

Figure 8-1   Visual analog scale for music/antianxiety study.

Concepts in Action *(continued)*

of most hospital satisfaction questionnaires and is generally regarded by both clinical staff and physicians as an important aspect of a patient's care. Nurses in this ICU overheard patient comments that they wished they could talk to their doctor more and that they had unanswered questions even after talking with their doctor. Their concerns formed the basis for a study that employed a quick, convenient data collection tool to maximize data capture.

Nurses created a simple label to place on the patient's Kardex. The label had a box for nurses to check when the physician spoke with the patient and family that day. There was a place for the nurse to indicate whether the patient felt that his or her questions had been answered and whether he or she was satisfied with the conversation. This label was filled out daily, beginning on the day the patient was admitted to the ICU until he or she was transferred to a medical–surgical unit.

Data Collection Challenges

This study was piloted for several weeks, but only a few of the labels were filled out. Primarily the study team was completing the labels. The team discussed this project at several staff meetings and their colleagues seemed to understand what needed to be done and pledged support.

Rest in the ICU: Using Instruments to Record Sound

Rest is considered an important aspect of recovery for all patients. There are many things in an ICU environment that can disturb rest. These ICU staff wanted to understand the factors in the ICU environment that interfere with a patient's ability to rest. They also wanted to determine what patients, their families, and nurses perceive as the main disturbances to a patient's ability to rest in the ICU.

A hospital safety professional was contacted for a sound meter, and sound samplings were taking at various periods and in various locations, inside and outside patient rooms, in the ICU. Perception questionnaires were developed and given to patients and their families and to ICU staff.

Data Collection Challenges

The sound meter did not provide continuous readings, and it was difficult to isolate individual sounds since this was a large (28-bed) ICU. It was difficult to provide a consistent, comparable assessment of each room, as there was a considerable amount of variability in each room environ-

(continues)

Concepts in Action *(continued)*

ment related to the type of equipment that was needed to treat the patient and the number of different clinicians and disciplines who needed to treat or interact with the patient. However, the results stimulated improvements. Although the first part of this study was aimed at identifying issues and not intervention, several changes were made. When a high noise level factor was identified—including loud shoes worn by one physician, irritating sounds from the garbage bin, and squeaky wheels on a cart—the source of the noise was identified, and staff intervened.

Preoperative and Postoperative Endotoxemia in Children With Congenital Heart Disease: Using Physiological Samples

Endotoxins can cause or worsen cardiac dysfunction in children with congenital heart disease. If endotoxin is found in this population of children, treatment can potentially lessen any cardiac dysfunction associated with the endotoxemia. This study sought to determine the incidence, clinical relevance, and magnitude of endotoxemia before and after surgical repair.

The researchers planned to measure the plasma levels of bacterial endotoxin or lipopolysaccharide (LPS) and lipopolysaccharide-binding protein (LBP), which increases in response to exposure to bacteria and their endotoxins. LBP is a plasma protein with a longer half-life than LPS. It was anticipated that measurement of both LPS and LBP would provide a good indicator of the prevalence of endotoxemia.

Blood samples were drawn prior to surgery and 1, 8, 24, 48, and 72 hours after completion of cardiopulmonary bypass.

Data Collection Challenges

Many factors can cause an inflammatory response, from something as simple as irritation from an intravenous catheter to the impact of the cardiopulmonary bypass machine and the cardiac surgery itself. Pro-

Concepts in Action *(continued)*

cedures can also affect the outcome of the test, such as leaving the blood in the test tube too long or not placing the specimen on ice. In this study, special attention was needed for the methods of blood sampling. Further complicating the study, the researchers discovered that all sealed test tubes for blood collection already have endotoxin in them but that a special brand that has low endotoxin levels could be purchased.

To address our blood sampling concerns, we obtained the preoperative sample from a newly placed central venous catheter. After each blood specimen draw, we immediately placed it on ice and walked it to the laboratory.

Summary

Data collection methods require careful thought. As you plan your study design, plan your data collection tools as well. Run your data collection plan by your colleagues who have been actively involved in research studies and get advice from experienced researchers. If drug trials are underway in your organization, an often untapped resource is the research coordinator for these industry trials. A large part of their job requires expertise in data collection, and they can likely provide you with good input on what may or may not work. Do not forget to talk with the front line staff—even if you are a front-line staff member. They can usually quickly give you feedback to make your data collection methods better, and involving them will win their commitment to collect data for your study. Pilot your data collection sheets to discover problems while collecting data on a small scale. Document your data collection methods carefully, and revise them as you find out what works and what does not. Good research conclusions depend on accurate data, and complete data depends on convenient, clear data-collection methods.

A Checklist for Evaluating Numbers in Research

_____ Power was calculated and reported and is greater than 85%.

_____ Descriptive statistics are reported for the sample; standard error is relatively small.

_____ The researchers tested for group equivalency on key characteristics, and a large p value (indicating *no* differences between groups) was reported.

_____ Measurement tools were reliable.

_____ Reliability statistics were reported and were within acceptable levels.

_____ P values were reported for all hypothesis tests, and those reported as statistically significant were less than 0.05.

_____ The right statistical tests were used for the research question and the level of measurement.

_____ Actual test statistics were reported, and effect sizes were large enough to be clinically meaningful.

_____ Confidence intervals were reported and represent an acceptable level of precision.

Part IV

Using Bedside Science in Practice

CHAPTER 9

Can We Use It?

In this chapter, you will learn to

- Evaluate the external validity of a research study
- Assess whether you can apply research findings to your practice
- Use a systematic approach to translate research findings into clinical practice
- Describe communication channels for effective practice change
- Strengthen the generalizability of your studies

Your manager brings you an article about a research study that re-sulted in the savings of several thousand dollars a month for an academic medical center pharmacy. The study—conducted in a large metropolitan center on the East Coast—reported on a change in processes that imposed restrictions on certain formulary drugs that residents could order independently. The findings were dramatic—a reduction in both errors and costs for the pharmacy and an improvement in patient outcomes. Your manager passes on the article with a note, "Let's try this here!"

The research does appear to be particularly well done. Controls were in place for extraneous variables. The sample size was more than adequate, and the measures used were automated and reli-able. You have some concerns, however, about whether you will be able to reap the same benefits for your facility. For example, yours is a small community hospital, and you have no residents. The hos-

pital is located in a rural area and is only about a fifth as big as the hospital reported in the study. Even if the procedures reported in the research were in place, simple mathematics shows that your savings will not be nearly as dramatic.

You worry about the costs that you might incur that are not financial. You have a relatively small number of physicians that routinely admit to your hospital, and you know most of them personally. You are not sure how experienced practitioners would respond to limitations on their prescribing authority and are concerned that putting too many restrictions on their practices would drive your medical staff to the larger medical center that is 50 miles away. You do not want to appear resistant to change but are feeling that perhaps your pharmacy should slow down and make a considered decision about whether the findings from another study can be applied to your situation.

Finding well-done, relevant research is not the end of the research evaluation process. Rather, effective evidence-based practice changes are dependent on finding credible results that can be applied effectively in your setting with a reasonable expectation of success. The application process depends in part on finding studies with strong external validity and in part on changing the way people think and act as a result of the studies. Both are important for a successful research-based change in practice.

ABOUT EXTERNAL VALIDITY

External validity is the link between *finding* knowledge through research and *using* knowledge in practice. Whether a research project can be used in your specific situation with your specific patients is a function of external validity. External validity refers to the ability to generalize the findings from a research study to other populations, places, and situations.

Obviously, research studies done in limited settings or with small, convenience samples may not generalize well to other populations. However, there are many reasons that external validity may be limited, even in large, multisite studies. Table 9-1 summarizes some of the identified threats to external validity, what they are, and how they can be controlled.

Two types of external validity exist: ecological and population. *Ecological* validity refers to findings that can be generalized to other settings. For example, a study has strong ecological validity if it is conducted in an acute-care setting in a tertiary-care center, and you want to apply the findings in a similar

Table 9-1 Common Threats to External Validity and Their Control

Threat	What It Is	How It Is Controlled
Selection effects	The way subjects are recruited and selected may limit generalization to all populations; for example, volunteers and compensated subjects may have motives that are different from the population in general.	Select samples randomly. Choose samples from real-world settings. Report descriptive data for subjects so that external validity can be objectively evaluated.
Refusal and attrition	Subjects may refuse to participate or drop out of a study in a way that introduces systematic bias; those that refuse may share some characteristic that would inform the study. As the proportion who do not participate increases, external validity decreases.	Limit the investment demands (time, effort, and discomfort) on subjects to improve participation. Report descriptive data for those who refuse to participate and those who do not complete the study to judge the impact on the generalization. Report overall refusal and attrition rates.
Setting bias	Settings that encourage research and agree to participate may introduce bias via shared characteristics; research-resistant organizations may not be represented at all.	Consider the characteristics of the setting when discussing generalization of the study to other organizations. Use random selection when possible.
Historical effects	The unique circumstances in which a study was conducted may exert an influence on the outcome.	Have replication of the study during different time periods. Consider the timing of the study when suggesting generalization of findings.

setting. Ecological validity is also evident if a study done in one geographic area can be generalized to other geographic areas. For example, studies conducted in Colorado might reasonably be generalized to other Western states at similar altitudes. *Population* validity means that a study done in one group of subjects can be applied to other subjects. A study has strong population validity if it was conducted on a population that has characteristics that are similar to your patients. Age, gender, ethnicity, or diagnoses are examples of characteristics that might limit external generalization. Subject groups that are more diverse generally have more external population validity; highly homogeneous subjects, on the other hand, have limited generalizability.

Although there are many considerations in the control of external validity, the strongest element is the sampling strategy. The sampling process determines whether subjects are representative of the larger population and whether they can reasonably be expected to represent all patients.

Unfortunately, many of the measures used to control internal validity—very tightly drawn inclusion and exclusion criteria, sample matching, and stratified random sampling, for example—make it difficult to maximize external validity. When samples become so homogeneous that most extraneous variables are controlled, they no longer represent the real world very well. Generating research that is generalizable, then, is created by a balance between control of internal validity and real-world sampling.

When you read a research study to determine whether it applies to your patients and your situation, focus on these key aspects:

1. How is the population defined? If the population characteristics sound like those of your patients, then the study may have generalizability to your practice.

2. Are there extraneous variables in your situation (or in the research situation) that could affect the outcome? For example, your region may have a high proportion of non–English-speaking patients or a larger proportion of older patients. On the other hand, there might be an extraneous variable that exerts no effect. The decision of whether a variable exerts an effect requires clinical judgment.

3. Is the setting one that reasonably approximates yours? If differences exist, they may not have any impact at all or may render the study virtually inapplicable.

4. Have the findings been replicated with a range of subjects in different settings? Continued testing of findings in multiple studies or in multiple sites increases the ability to transfer results to more diverse situations. Replication is both a hallmark of scholarly work and a source of increased confidence in the findings. Multisite studies provide some of the strongest evidence for both generalizability and support for practice change.

Where to Look for Information About External Validity

External validity is rarely directly addressed in a research study. The reader's responsibility is to determine whether the subjects, setting, and procedures are similar enough to expect the findings to apply to their specific situation. However, some specific elements of the report can help the reader make that assessment.

- Look for an identification of the population in the introduction, the research question, or within the sampling strategy. Along with a specific description of the population, inclusion and exclusion criteria can help you determine whether the patients will reasonably approximate yours. Review tables that describe the specific characteristics of the final sample to decide whether they resemble your patients closely enough that you could expect the findings to generalize well.

- The research question may also indicate the setting, although a generic description of the geographic region is generally a part of the introduction to the study. If not included early in the study, then a description of the type of setting (e.g., long-term care, acute care, ambulatory settings) and the geographic location (e.g., a metropolitan area in the south, a rural setting in the Midwest) should precede the results. It may be specifically labeled "setting." These are critical elements of the study and should be explicitly noted. If they are not, you cannot assume that the results will apply to your practice.

- Authors will many times explicitly discuss external validity in the discussion and conclusion sections. Researchers may suggest other patients and settings in which the results could be expected to apply. There may be a specific section of the discussion in which generalizability—or its lack—is discussed. Even so, the final responsibility for determining applicability is your judgment and knowledge of your patients.

As you read, ask yourself whether the sample and environment of the study are similar enough to your conditions that you could reasonably expect the results to be applied successfully. If the defined population and environment are considerably different from yours, then results that were achieved in the study may not be accomplished in your situation.

How similar do the study specifics have to be to yours for successful generalization? Do not expect to find studies that have exactly the same patient mix in an identical situation. You need to use your critical judgment to evaluate whether the results of a study should be used in your practice. Although the authors might suggest extensions of the study or potential sites for application, the final responsibility lies with the reader to decide whether a study can be translated from research into reality.

Hitting the Stacks

Wong, Ghaleb, Franklin, and Barer (2004) noted that their findings about the incidence and nature of dosing errors in pediatric medications may not apply in settings other then Great Britain, where the study was conducted. "The incidence of medication errors is likely to vary depending on the setting in which the research was conducted. . . . In UK hospitals, clinicians usually prescribe using a pro-forma drug chart, which is also used to document drug administration. . . . In US hospitals, clinicians traditionally prescribe on a blank 'doctor's order' sheet, on which all the doctors' orders are written. . . . In European hospitals, clinicians prescribe medications in a section of the patient's medical notes with other instructions to nurses. . . . Considering the above differences, the epidemiology, causes of errors and potential solutions are likely to be different than those presented here."

Bagley et al. (2005) similarly noted that their sampling strategy—specifically, inclusion criteria—seriously limited the generalizability of a negative finding relative to use of the Oswestry Standing Frame for patients after stroke. Although the authors found that the standing frame was not an effective intervention in this study, they noted several reasons why this may not apply to most patients. "The principal study inclusion criterion (patients who were unable to stand upright without the assistance of two therapists) necessarily led to a majority group (65%) of stroke patients with large cortical lesions. These patients have a poor prognosis for recovery of function. Therefore, while this study was attempting to identify a treatment with the potential to benefit patients with severe stroke disability, functional improvements for these patients might be difficult to achieve. . . . The role of supported standing as a treatment strategy for patients able to stand independently after stroke remains uncertain."

Wong, I.C., A.G. Maisoon, B.D. Franklin, and N. Barber. 2004. Incidence and nature of dosing errors in paediatric medications: A systematic review. *Drug Safety* 27: 661–70.

Bagley, P., M. Hudson, A. Forster, J. Smith, and J. Young. 2005. A randomized trial evaluation of the Oswestry Standing Frame for patients after stroke. *Clinical Rehabilitation* 19: 354–64.

APPLICATION OF BEDSIDE SCIENCE PROJECTS
TO THE REAL WORLD

The concern with external validity is less important for your internal bedside science projects. When a research project is conducted in the very situation it is expected to address—and with the group of patients of particular interest—then application is more straightforward. The concern with specific bedside science projects is not *whether* the findings should be applied but *how* that application will be accomplished. This is more complicated than it might appear. Although research is very systematic and logical, complex organizational systems are not. It is still reasonable to use a logical, stepwise approach—but do not expect that change will occur in a logical way. Effort, focus, and communication skills are critical for a successful transition.

Many challenges are inherent in trying to translate research into practice. There may be a lack of adequate preparation for reading and using research among staff, or research skills may be unused and rusty. Broader organizational factors—such as lack of manager support, inadequate resources, or limited time—may also play a role in preventing the quick uptake of research results. More insidious barriers—for example, a lack of belief in the value of research, or a change-resistant culture—may hinder utilization.

Winch, Henderson, and Creedy (2005) propose a model for fitting research findings into practice. Called the "Read, Think, Do!" method, this process provides an approach for influencing clinical decision making and practice change. The plan recognizes that social and cultural change may be as necessary as the empirical evidence for the uptake of research findings. This approach acknowledges the complexity of translating research into practice and advocates a three-step process to create change:

1. *Read:* This step involves gaining access to research findings that will provide an empirical basis for a change in practice.

2. *Think:* The clinician then applies critical thought about the relevance of the study for their practice and whether the results can be generalized intact or in some modified form.

3. *Do:* The final step involves organizing the practice change within the local culture, with an attention to the dynamics of the social and belief changes that may be needed.

Clearly, the third step is the most challenging. The bedside scientist can, however, use a systematic approach to managing social and cultural change. Given that the impetus for the research likely arose from a practice problem identified by clinicians, it is reasonable that staff should be involved in planning and undertaking the change. When individuals are involved in decisions

Another Way to Look at External Validity

External validity is enhanced by careful sampling and replication but is still not assured for a specific population and setting. Deciding whether results with one group of patients in one setting will apply to yours is up to you. Other variables that exist in your situation—but that were not in the study—may mean that you can use the results, but they will not work the same.

I have had this experience most often when trying to translate the pictures out of "beautiful house" magazines to my own home. Trying to picture how the house will look from a paint chip or from a couple of square feet of shingle is anything but precise. I have tried driving around neighborhoods looking at different combinations, buying innumerable pints of paint to draw a swathe across the front, and coloring in digital photos on my computer. It seems, however, that no matter what I have done to project what my house will look like it never quite turns out the way I expect.

Sometimes the difference is due to the small sample size—it really is hard to picture how a couple of inches of paint will look when it covers a three-dimensional object as big as a house. Sometimes the difference is due to things in my neighborhood that others might not have—the 50-foot elm next door that drops brown branches year round on our green roof or the way the sun bounces off our windows during the day. There is also a real potential that the difference in the way my house looks and the way the ones in the magazine look is poor execution—home repair is not my strength.

The differences may be so big that the look of it never really feels right, and I look forward to a chance to redo it again. Other times, the differences do not have a real impact on the overall look of it, and I choose to adopt the new look as it works for my house.

Of course, no house in a magazine ever looked like my house to begin with, and no study will every have a sample and setting that look exactly like your patients and your environment. It is your clinical judgment, combined with a critical eye on the design of the research, that helps you determine whether concerns about the differences are outweighed by the potential for a meaningful change in clinical practice.

about implementation, they are more likely to adopt the change. Those who have participated in specific change planning will be more committed to its success. There are other advantages to gaining staff input into a change. Facilitated discussions about the change in staff meetings or via other communication methods (e-mail, surveys) may also bring to light legitimate barriers to overcome as well as creative solutions.

A general approach is to devise a protocol for change based on the research results and then allow time for review and input about the specifics of the protocol. Feedback should be solicited from the clinicians expected to implement the practice change as well as from those who will be indirectly affected by the change or whose patients may be affected by the change. Explore concerns carefully, and assume they are legitimate. Knowing these up front may present an opportunity to avoid problems during implementation. Be sure to consider the impact on other departments and the fact that their resources may be affected as well.

From the Mouths of Bedside Scientists: How Clinicians Talk About Research in Practice

What do you look for in finding a study to apply to your practice?

I look for studies that examine those things that I may be interested in implementing. This includes studies that were done years ago or those that are just entering the trial phase. I look for the ease of introducing the new technique and how much backing this change will have. Also, I look for studies that have been replicated numerous times and see the conditions in which they were performed. If all of these items come together, then I go about implementation.

When I look for a study to apply to my practice, I first look for a similar demographic population, with similar practices to mine. For example, when looking at a study to help support a change in treatment for a given patient population, I first look for studies from hospitals of similar size, patient population, and practice patterns to try and minimize variables that might not be mentioned in the study but that could affect the results.

How is empirical evidence used to change practice?

Empirical evidence should be used continuously to change practice for the better. It is important in several respects. Empirical evidence provides us with guidance regarding which parts of current practice need modification or improvement. Evidence can also help us use resources in a more effective manner. Evidence gives practitioners the ethical guidelines for treating their patients. Empirical results also give us ideas for new studies because it seems every time the evidence provides us with an answer, it gives us more questions as well.

Specific assignments should be given to those in leadership positions to assure that structural, procedural, material, and financial resources will be available to support the change in practice. Many a practice change has floundered because inadequate resources were applied to assure its success.

This involvement of staff in the practice change process encourages a sense of ownership for the change. Even with extensive input and staff planning, some specific steps must be taken to assure that the change is successful. Using appropriate channels for the change and communication—both interpersonal and organizational—is essential for success.

Use Appropriate Channels for Change

Organizations have expected processes that must be used to organize and implement change. Check with leadership to determine where to start with a change and how to assure that all organizational requirements are met. Often, practice changes are initiated and guided by the quality department or a research department. A practice council—a group of staff level clinicians that manage decisions about clinical practice—may have specific review and reporting procedures. Generally, clinical practice change projects are documented on specific records or within particular software systems to demonstrate the presence of research-based improvements for regulatory and credentialing agencies. The primary considerations are (1) policies governing how clinical practice changes are approved; (2) groups that should be apprised of the progress and who will monitor the success of the change; and (3) records of the change that must be kept as documentation of the efforts. Clarify these expectations before starting the change plan. Make sure that communication is a key focus of the effort.

Internal Communication Channels

Multiple internal communication channels can be used to broadly disseminate a change in practice. Some common methods include the following:

1. Staff meetings
2. Unit-based practice councils
3. Organizationally based practice councils
4. Quality councils
5. E-mail dissemination to employees
6. Newsletters
7. Informational flyers

> ## For more depth and detail, try these resources:
>
> Burkiewicz, J.S., and D.P. Zgarrick. 2005. Evidence-based practice by pharmacists: Utilization and barriers. *The Annals of Pharmacotherapy* 39: 1214–9.
>
> Ferguson, L. 2004. External validity, generalizability, and knowledge utilization. *Journal of Nursing Scholarship* 36: 16–22.
>
> Hoagwood, K.E., and B.J. Burns. 2005. Evidence-based practice, part II: Effecting change. *Child and Adolescent Psychiatric Clinics of North America* 14: xv–xvii.
>
> Matcher, D.B., E.V. Westermann-Clar, D.C. McCrory, M. Patwardhan, G. Samsa, S. Kulasingam, E. Myers, A. Sarria-Santameria, A. Lee, R. Gray, and K. Liu. 2004. Dissemination of evidence-based practice center reports. *Annals of Internal Medicine* 142(12 Pt. 2): 1120–5.
>
> Rothwell, P.M. 2005. External validity of randomized controlled trials: "To whom do the results of this trial apply?" *Lancet* 365: 82–94.
>
> Rycroft-Malone, J., G. Harvey, K. Seers, A. Kitson, B. McCormack, and A. Titchen. 2004. An exploration of the factors that influence the implementation of evidence into practice. *Journal of Clinical Nursing* 13: 913–24.
>
> Scalzitti, D.A. 2001. Evidence-based guidelines: Application to clinical practice. *Physical Therapy* 81: 1622–8.
>
> Sudsawad, P. 2005. A conceptual framework to increase usability of outcome research for evidence-based practice. *The American Journal of Occupational Therapy* 59: 351–5.
>
> Winch, S., A. Henderson, and D. Creedy. 2005. Read, think, do! A method for fitting research evidence into practice. *Journal of Advanced Nursing* 50: 20–6.

8. Postings on bulletin boards and in break rooms

9. Communication logs or electronic discussion boards

This is a common but not exhaustive list of communication channels available for practice change. Communication will be most effective when multiple methods are used. Not all employees will be reached with a single approach; multiple communication channels, as well as multiple ways that the message can be structured, can increase the chance that the change will reach the clinicians who are expected to make it successful.

Strengthen the External Validity of Your Studies

It is difficult to achieve strong external validity with a convenience sample. Without multiple sites, multiple studies, and access to large, heterogeneous populations, it is rare that a bedside science project will have broad generalizability. That does not mean that you cannot take steps to maximize the applicability of your study across units in your organization or to similar units in other organizations:

- Use an element of randomness in your sample selection, even if it is as simple as flipping a coin to determine who is asked to be in the study.
- Limit inclusion and exclusion criteria to those that are critical for control of a major extraneous variable that can be assumed to exert an effect.
- Try to gain as much diversity as possible in the sample by using multiple units, different time frames, and procedures that are ethnically inclusive.
- Replicate a small study several times instead of attempting to carry out one large study. The increasing sample size achieved by several small studies adds diversity to the sample and power to the study.
- Account for potential threats to external validity such as historical events, treatment effects, and researcher bias in your write-up.

Changing Policies and Procedures

Communicating a change with multiple channels will help initiate the change, but continuing success of the change will depend on a permanent record describing the change in practice and transforming it from "new procedure" to "established procedure." This requires that relevant policies and procedures are developed, disseminated, and adopted in permanent form. Many organizations have a paper policy manual, or policies and procedures may be electronically stored. Leaders can help you identify how to go about writing, gaining approval for, and ensuring adoption of an evidence-based practice change.

SUMMARY

Evidence-based practice is focused on finding appropriate evidence and creating an empirically based change in practice. This requires that you are able to determine critically whether a study has external validity—that is, whether the study can be applied to your specific patients and situation. Your evaluation of the applicability of the study is the most important step in this process.

After it has been determined that a change is appropriate, then many clinicians should be consulted about the specific nature of the change in practice and the plan for its implementation. Involvement will encourage ownership of the change. Social and cultural considerations should guide the successful change process. Although many barriers exist for the transformation from research to reality, overcoming the challenge offers tremendous rewards.

Concepts in Action

Internal practice-based studies are often the most useful for bedside scientists, as they answer very specific questions and there is no concern about the transferability of findings from an unfamiliar setting or population. These studies may arise from quality-improvement questions focused on process improvement, but use a systematic review of the literature and empirical data to answer the question. As such, these studies overlap both applied studies and research.

The bedside scientist may find their first exposure to the design and conduct of research projects through service on a quality improvement team. As this study illustrates, a systematic approach, a thorough literature review, and data collection distinguish these studies from pure process improvement efforts. The bedside scientist will do well to volunteer for a quality improvement study as a way to learn about practice-based research projects and the challenges of a systematic data analysis process.

What were the questions studied in this bedside project?
What is causing an increase in hypoglycemia-related insulin notification reports? How can nurses get comfortable with new insulin and diabetes management orders in our inpatient population?

Why was this research question important?
Patients who are admitted with diabetes and require insulin are becoming a quickly growing percentage of many hospital's cases. Changes in the types of insulin that are available and in the expectations for the care of patients with diabetes have required modification in long-standing clinical practice. The American Association of Clinical Endocrinologists introduced a position statement in December of 2003 discussing the importance of tight glycemic control and of the relationship between inpatient hyperglycemia and adverse outcomes. The American Diabetes Association released a statement in September of 2004 related to carbohydrates and their role in

(continues)

Concepts in Action *(continued)*

the prevention and management of diabetes. These statements motivated a change in approach toward inpatient diabetes management.

Clinicians in this mountain-state, tertiary-care hospital recognized the need for new standards of practice for insulin-dependent diabetics and formed a team to research best practice and recommend change. The standard practice of generic sliding scale insulin protocols using regular insulin and the timing of blood sugar checks and insulin administration needed to be changed. All of the new procedures needed to be based on sound evidence.

In order to obtain tighter glycemic control in the inpatient population, analogue insulin replaced regular insulin on the hospital's sliding scale protocol. Some medical staff began ordering carbohydrate counting and correction factors for inpatients who have diabetes and are able to eat. These are patients who tend to be admitted to the medical–surgical, orthopedic, oncology, and bone marrow transplant units.

The fact that the goal was to keep tighter control on hyperglycemia in the hospital led to the risk of patients becoming hypoglycemic. If a patient becomes hypoglycemic, he or she could become unconscious, possibly leading to an arrest situation. As the practice changes were initiated, these events became very important to prevent.

This research question was first introduced in the nutrition support committee, which is a subcommittee of the pharmacy and therapeutics committee. Nutritionists, physicians, and diabetes educators were being paged frequently by the nursing staff regarding carbohydrate counting orders and how to interpret them. This was reinforced by the pharmacy reporting an increase in medication errors related to insulin administration.

Who was involved on the research team?

This team was truly multidisciplinary. Physicians from endocrinology and medicine, registered dietitians, nursing education, pharmacy, nursing, diabetes management, and quality management all took part in this process. It was directed by the quality management department, and the chairperson of this committee was a patient care director.

What were the methods that were planned?

The team's work focused on developing a plan for education of the staff regarding best practice and changes in procedures. Two members of the team undertook a literature search. The articles were mainly first-tier studies; the search did not include qualitative studies. The team also incorporated the position statements of both the American Diabetes

Concepts in Action *(continued)*

Association and the American Association of Clinical Endocrinologists related to the benefits of tight glycemic control in the hospital. They offered recommendations for obtaining good glycemic control while controlling the risks of hypoglycemia. Very little information was found on carbohydrate counting in the inpatient setting. Several articles addressed this topic in an outpatient setting, however. These articles were evaluated by many of the committee members and were used to form a basis for recommendations for practice change and staff development.

Because of the severity of insulin-related hypoglycemia events, the committee members chose a systematic study design frequently used in quality studies, called the Plan, Do, Study, Act model. This approach has the advantage of speed while maintaining a rigorous approach to problem solving.

Working from the Plan, Do, Study, Act approach, three goals were identified: to decrease the number of insulin-related hypoglycemia events, to increase nurse knowledge of types and actions of insulin, and to educate staff nurses on carbohydrate counting in the inpatient setting.

Outcome Measures

The next question was this: "What indicators will tell us if this change is an improvement?" The answer was threefold. The first was an expected decrease in the number of notification reports that are related to the delivery of insulin, resulting in hypoglycemia. The second was an increase in nurses understanding the carbohydrate counting orders, as evidenced by a decrease in pages to nutritional services, the ordering physician, and diabetes services. Finally, it was expected that increased patient education would improve patients notifying the nurse that their meal has arrived.

The Protocol for Change

Many recommendations were quickly developed, based on the literature review, the guidelines in the position statements, and the professional input of team members. Intervention began within the first month of the project. The team divided the project into phase I and phase II. Phase I was an educational intervention with the aim of bringing everyone up to date on the latest evidence for this practice. Phase II focused on carbohydrate counting and the correction factors used.

In phase I, education was developed around the term "Check, Dose, Eat." Education regarding types of insulin and their onset, peak, and duration was distributed to each nursing unit in the form of posters and

(continues)

Concepts in Action *(continued)*

flyers. One poster was formulated by the pharmacy department and included all of the evidence-based information, along with a picture of each vial used in the hospital. These posters were hung in each medication room on the affected units. The other posters and flyers focused on how to prevent hypoglycemia in patients who have analogue (rapid-acting) insulin ordered. This education was accomplished through a combination of inservice and staff meetings.

Staff was taught to educate patients to notify nursing when their meal trays arrive. Staff would then check their blood sugar with the food present, and patients would receive any needed insulin at the same time that they were eating. Certain units, where patients sometimes struggle to keep their food down after they consume it, were educated to the fact that the patient's insulin can be given within 15 minutes after they finish their meal. This phase included Food and Nutrition Services placing a sticky note on the outer tray of all patients receiving diabetic diets to further educate the patient to notify their nurse. This note, in both English and Spanish, has increased patient compliance and understanding of the insulin administration process (Figure 9-1). The largest change of practice for the nursing staff was the timing of blood sugar checks; these were done at times that were much different than current practice.

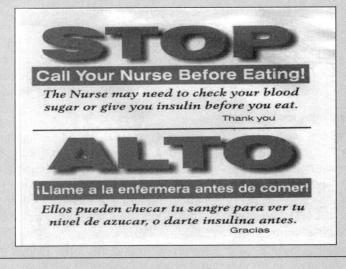

Figure 9-1   Patient education note for meal trays.

Concepts in Action *(continued)*

Phase II focused on the carbohydrate counting and the correction factors that the team endocrinologist had developed. The diabetes management team again provided inservice to all the affected departments and gave many examples of different correction factors. The staff was provided with carbohydrate counting calculation cards with the formulas and examples for use by nursing personnel (Figure 9-2). These hang with the staff's ID badge and provide a quick reference for staff. Nutrition services was involved in this phase and provided a complete list of menu items and the grams of carbohydrates for each item. This was provided to all managers and posted in each patient room and the medication room to ensure consistency in the calculations required with carbohydrate counting.

Front of Card	Back of Card
Determining the amount of insulin to give your carbohydrate counting patient	**Example:** BGG = 100 GCF = 1 unit/25 mg/dL CCF = 1 unit/30 gm CHO Current BG = 223mg/dL
Abbreviations: Blood Glucose Goal: BGG Glucose Correction Factor: GCF Carbohydrate Correction Factor: CCF	223 − 100 = 123(mg/dL)/25 = 4.92 units (5 units)
Equation: **Current blood glucose − BGG =** **___ / GCF = ___ # units**	Total number of grams of carbs on tray = 72 gm 72gm/30 gm = 2.4 units (2 units)
Add up number of grams of carbs on patient's tray	5 units + 2 units = 7 units Novalog
Total grams of carbs / CCF = **____ # units**	
Add BG units + CCF units = **Total units of Novalog**	

Figure 9-2 Carbohydrate counting card for nurse reference.

Concepts in Action *(continued)*

Results

Data related to notification reports were collected by the medication safety pharmacist on the team. Information from the two quarters before the intervention took place was compared with the two quarters after education took place, but showed little change. During this time, the percentage of patients admitted who had received at least one dose of insulin as an inpatient increased from 6.8% and 7.0% in third and fourth quarters of 2004 to 7.4% and 7.2% in the first and second quarter of 2005. Despite these increases in volumes, the actual number of notification reports stayed steady.

A short survey was distributed to the staff nurses of two of the units to which this education was offered. The questions asked the nurse's comfort level with carbohydrate counting before and after the education, and indeed, the reported comfort level rose from an average of 1.43 to an average of 2.35 on a scale of 0 to 3. Survey responses also indicated that 85% of nurses found the carbohydrate calculation card helpful. Additionally, the survey asked whether nurses felt that patients attained better glucose levels after the insulin education, and the vast majority of answers were positive.

What were the challenges that were faced?

This project faced challenges at the beginning because there was so little evidence to act on. Carbohydrate counting in an inpatient setting had not been documented as having been attempted at any other inpatient facility before this point. Because there was no proven practice that indicated the benefit of this practice in the inpatient setting, there were concerns about patient safety from nursing and pharmacy leadership. The research studies provided by the literature search, however, convinced the team and clinical decision makers that tight glycemic control, whether obtained with carbohydrate counting or any other means, should be the clinical goal.

Staff nurses were very quick to buy into phase I of the project. There was an almost immediate shift to blood sugars being obtained and insulin administered at the time that patient's received their meals, rather than 30 to 60 minutes before that. There was a little more resistance to the carbohydrate counting procedure, apparently because of its com-

Concepts in Action *(continued)*

plexity. The staff was given some tools to simplify the process, specifically calculation cards that explain the equations involved in carbohydrate counting. The staff still needed extensive training, but the outcome of decreasing calls to the attending physician was achieved.

It became evident as notification reports relating to hypoglycemia were nearly unchanged that there was another aspect of insulin delivery involved. Difficulties existed in retrieving accurate data about notification reports from a computer system, which may have skewed the results. A change in focus was proposed, and the group decided to pursue evidence related to the insulin drip protocol and the prospect of changing to a "multiplier"-based insulin drip protocol to increase control of blood sugars.

How was this study used?

This project was introduced throughout the adult units of the hospital at the same time. With the education in place and the practice changes implemented, the group continues to meet and discuss some practical issues regarding implementation and documentation. At this point, documentation of glucose levels, insulin given, carbohydrates consumed, and correction factors is all documented in multiple places. The group is now working with the information technology department to build a screen in our computer documentation where all of this information can be charted in a flow sheet.

The team continues to look at data regarding the goal of tighter glycemic control. The lab has pulled blood glucose values for the four quarters of the study and analysis focused on whether patients' blood sugars are falling into a smaller and healthier range.

How will it be communicated internally and to larger audiences?

Data from this team are monitored and reported to the nutrition support committee and pharmacy and therapeutics committee, usually every month or two. The patient care director who chaired this committee also shared information at the director and senior management level in their monthly meetings. It was also accepted and will be presented as a poster presentation at a medical surgical nursing conference.

Contributed by Julie Jones, Presbyterian/St. Luke's Medical Center, Denver, CO.

A Checklist for Evaluating Generalizability of Research

_____ The population in the study is similar to the patients you work with in general.

_____ The sample was selected randomly, and thus, it can be assumed to be representative.

_____ The descriptive statistics for the sample reveal a heterogeneous group.

_____ The setting for the study is similar to yours in key characteristics such as level of care, type of unit, and geographic locale.

_____ Extraneous variables in your setting are accounted for in the study.

_____ The authors controlled for the major threats to external validity—that is, historical events, treatment effects, and researcher effects.

_____ The inclusion and exclusion criteria are not so strict that the sample is artificial and cannot translate to the real world.

_____ The study has been replicated in different settings and with different subjects or in multiple sites.

CHAPTER 10

Finding Evidence in Words

In this chapter, you will learn to

- Identify research questions that are appropriately answered with survey and qualitative methods
- Decide on a sampling strategy for a survey or qualitative study
- Design a survey or questionnaire and test its reliability and validity
- Describe how survey and qualitative data are analyzed
- Apply the results from survey and qualitative studies to evidence-based practice
- Strengthen your survey and qualitative designs

You are feeling pretty good about your ability to evaluate a research study—particularly randomized trials. After all, you have been a key member of two systematic review teams and have helped to develop and communicate evidence-based changes in practice. Currently, you are helping a team in the emergency department, charged with determining best practice for patients who present with chest pain. You have reached a point in the team's work, however, where questions are raised that cannot be answered with numbers. What is it that makes one patient more compliant with the postdischarge plan than another? How does the family create demands on the staff that are unrelated to direct patient care? Why do some patients wait so long before coming in for treatment? Do providers have different attitudes about women with chest pain? As you address the clinical practices that are linked to better outcomes, you are finding gaps in the knowledge relative to the perceptual side of health care. It seems that those perceptions and attitudes—of both patients and staff—seem to give rise to some of the variations in practice that ultimately affect care.

The team decides to collect data directly from those who are most involved in the process—the patients and the emergency department staff. The team starts with a basic outline of the major questions that need to be answered and quickly realizes that a simple questionnaire will not capture all of the information needed. Some of the questions—especially those that start with "why?"—need to be explored rather than recorded. After writing specific items for each of the questions, the final survey is a bit of a mixed bag—some forced-choice items, some scales, and some open-ended questions. The team decides to write some general inclusion criteria for the sample but otherwise will collect data from anyone who is willing.

A pilot test of the instrument shows you that the open-ended questions are not being answered when the subject has to write the answers out for you. It is also clear that a couple of the questions are confusing and that you have written the survey at too high of a reading level. The questionnaire is revised, and the team makes the tough decision that the open-ended questions will need to be answered with interviews. You decide to limit those to just a few carefully chosen subjects.

Data collection is a lot of work, but it pays off. You have found that attitudes and perceptions do fill in many of the knowledge gaps, sometimes with surprising information. Who knew that the anxiety of families is a key reason for readmissions and that women rationalize away subtle signs of heart attacks more than men? Who knew that the patients in your emergency department rated fear a higher distress to them than pain? Armed with the information from the study, your team is able to combine science and compassion to achieve better outcomes for your patients.

Sometimes gaps exist in our clinical expertise that are unrelated to easily quantifiable events. Health care is a service that is delivered to and by people, and this human aspect of clinical practice is part of what draws us to be caregivers. There are also variables that need study in health care that cannot be manipulated, for either physiologic or ethical reasons. For these, collecting data in words may be the most effective way to find key information for clinical practice. These methods—analysis of perceptions, attitudes, or knowledge—generally fall into two categories: survey methods and qualitative research.

Survey methods can fall on the border between quantitative and qualitative research. Although surveys generally capture information that is subjective in nature, they often possess strong reliability and produce measurable outcomes. Measuring intelligence or depression, for example, translates a very subjective characteristic into a quantifiable value, but does so in a highly structured and systematic way.

Some surveys, however, produce more subjective information, particularly open-ended survey questions. Qualitative research, on the other hand, is solely collected through observation and interaction, and these data are collected as notes or transcripts.

Even though survey and qualitative research are focused on collecting a different type of data, the rules for doing good research do not change because of it. A systematic approach, internal validity, control of bias, and enhancement of transferability are all-important goals, regardless of the research method. The ways that these are *achieved* differ, as does the way the results are used in clinical practice.

WHAT IS SURVEY RESEARCH?

Survey methods are a popular way of gathering descriptive information about a population. A researcher can reach a large sample in an efficient manner using survey methods. A survey method is an approach in which a systematic measurement instrument is used to gather information directly from subjects about their experiences, behaviors, attitudes, or perceptions. Survey methods generally depend on the reports of the subjects themselves and differ from other measurement methods in that an objective researcher is not gathering the data. Rather, the subjects themselves are judging and reporting their own responses.

Survey research blends some of the characteristics of quantitative research with characteristics of more subjective qualitative methods. As such, the survey researcher needs skills for both quantitative and qualitative design and analysis. Numbers may be used to describe the responses of subjects, in scale scores, measurements, or words. A systematic approach and quantitative analysis of reliability, validity, and statistical conclusions are characteristic of survey research.

WHAT IS QUALITATIVE RESEARCH?

Qualitative methods are based on observation and interaction and capture, in detail, the nature of something significant in the social world of people. As a rule, the findings are descriptive and do not attempt to measure relationships or determine effects. This group of methods is tied to a specific context and thus is not conducted in controlled settings such as laboratories. Rather, qualitative studies are applied studies, occurring in the environment where the subject "lives," in their world rather than the researcher's. Because of this close tie to a specific environment, qualitative research is not generalizable in the traditional sense. Transferability of results is limited to those settings and patients that are very similar to those in the study.

Qualitative research differs from quantitative designs in other fundamental ways. In general—in contrast to the detailed plans set out for experiments—qualitative designs are emergent. This means that the subjects, content of questions, and even data collection methods may change as the study progresses. The researcher admits to their biases but otherwise is immersed in the study rather than objectively blinded to the details. In fact, the researcher *is* the data collection instrument, and thus, the reliability and validity of results are based most centrally on their skills. Even data analysis is an emergent and

---

Another Way to Look at It

Scientists often have trouble incorporating the results of survey and qualitative designs into evidence-based practice guidelines because the traditional standards for evaluating a research study do not apply. However, data gathered about the more subjective, human side of health care can be very useful in assuring that patients achieve the outcomes *they* desire, rather than the ones we define for them. The definition of evidence-based practice advanced in this book is "practice based on the best available evidence combined with the patient's preferences." In general, the ways we find out about the patient's preferences are through more subjective data collection methods and analysis based on words.

This has been a key understanding for me based on my own very human experience with the health care system as a patient. When I was 9 years old, I had my appendix removed. Now, I will not give away my age by telling you the year, but suffice it to say that I had a *routine* 7-day hospital stay, a 6-inch incision, and anesthesia delivered as a gas through a face mask. The gas was sickeningly sweet, and I threw up in the mask. I will never forget the panicky feeling of being afraid that I was going to aspirate while I was simultaneously going under anesthesia.

Years later, I needed surgery that required anesthesia. By this time, the anesthesia came in an intravenous drip. I had learned that the surgical procedure could result in postoperative pain, that there were risks of complications, and that it would likely take me weeks to recover. None

ongoing process, as new data are constantly compared with existing data and analyzed simultaneously with data collection.

Qualitative research tends to be holistic, considering and incorporating all effects into the study results rather than attempting to control them. It can be seen from even the most basic characteristics that qualitative research requires a completely different skill set than experimental research. It answers research questions that are focused on the human experience rather than the physiological one.

THE USE OF SURVEY AND QUALITATIVE DESIGNS AS EVIDENCE

Many scientists find it difficult to evaluate the characteristics of survey and qualitative designs, as traditional standards for quantitative research are difficult to apply. The nature of survey and qualitative research is fundamentally different. Conducting these types of studies requires a basic shift in the way that we think about the nature and importance of evidence.

Another Way to Look at It *(continued)*

of that, however, was my focus the evening before the surgery—all I could think of was that moment when they would put a mask over my face and put me to sleep.

When the anesthesiologist visited me, she did all of the things you would expect—checked my lab results, my vital signs, and my neurological condition. She collected all of the right health history and quantitative information. Then she asked me something I did not expect (although this one question helped her to understand how best to care for me): "What is it about this procedure that scares you the most?" It gave me the opportunity to tell her about my "fear of the mask," about my childhood experience, about the thing I dreaded more than the pain or complications or lengthy recovery. With one sentence from her—"Then I'll just wait till you are good and asleep to put the mask on you"—a dreadful experience was changed to one that was surprisingly uneventful.

That anesthesiologist used the best quantitative evidence available to her and combined it with qualitative evidence to create a health care experience that was both physiologically sound and compassionate. Evidence-based practice is about more than numbers and measures and randomized trials. It is about remembering that, at its most fundamental, health care is about people—people that we see when they are at their most frightened, frail, and vulnerable. Using all the available evidence to improve their lives— whether numbers or words—is what good bedside scientists accomplish.

That is not to say that survey and qualitative data cannot be useful in clinical practice. In fact, it is often the human side of health care that can make the difference between a good outcome and a poor one. The way we define quality of life, for example, is difficult to measure with traditional scientific methods, and yet no one would argue its importance in determining acceptable outcomes for patients. Through qualitative and survey research methods, we can gain richer insight into the lived experiences of our patients and our colleagues and learn ways to support and explain therapeutic effects better. Qualitative research is often the starting point for building mental models about cause and effect that can later be tested using quantitative techniques.

Survey methods may provide clinical practitioners with information about attitudes or values, levels of knowledge or experience, current practices, or characteristics of specific patients. Standardized instruments are often used to determine levels of satisfaction and to measure outcomes such as functionality or quality of life.

The key to applying survey and qualitative findings as evidence is to use *method-appropriate* standards for their evaluation. Standards do exist for evaluating the validity of both survey designs and qualitative results. When good studies are found, the results should be used to fill gaps in knowledge that are rooted in the belief systems, values, perceptions, or social interactions of patients and caregivers.

Although survey and qualitative research findings are considered less reliable evidence when compared with quantitative counterparts, well-done survey and qualitative designs can be useful as evidence. Using survey and qualitative research findings requires more than a methodologic change, however; it requires a fundamental change in the way we think about research, truth, and the role of scientific findings in practice.

As in other types of research, a key step is formulation of a focused research question. The research question will frame the problem in such a way that it can be linked to a specific research design. Research questions that are best answered with survey or qualitative methods often begin with the words *why* or *how*. When the research question is focused, the researcher must then decide whether it is best answered with survey or qualitative methods or a combination of the two. Each has different procedures, characteristics, strengths, and limitations. Matching the design to the research question is a key step to arrive at useful, valid answers.

SURVEY RESEARCH

Survey designs are probably the most common research method. Survey research uses an instrument to collect data directly from respondents to answer specific research questions. Surveys allow access to large numbers of subjects with relative efficiency and enable the collection of data about attitudes, perceptions, and other less observable characteristics. It is challenging, however, to create a valid and reliable survey and to capture a representative sample.

Surveys can be descriptive or explanatory. Descriptive surveys evaluate the distribution of characteristics, attitudes, opinions, feelings, or experiences within a population. These may be specific to a single sample or intended for generalization to larger groups. Explanatory surveys attempt to examine relationships among variables and explain how these variables are related to each other. Both types of surveys require access to large, representative samples and measurement with an instrument that minimizes measurement error.

Sampling Strategies

The best survey samples are determined as they are in quantitative research—through large, randomly drawn samples from carefully defined populations. Although survey results are intended to be descriptive, a careful sampling strategy can enhance transferability of the results to larger populations. The sample should represent the population in its diversity; very homogeneous samples make for less external validity. As in experimental designs, sampling error should be minimized through objective inclusion criteria, the use of exclusion criteria, and probability sampling methods.

A key consideration in survey research is the response rate. Depending on the data collection methods, high response rates may be difficult to obtain. Telephone surveys generally have the lowest response rates, whereas higher response rates can be expected with web-based surveys. In general, if it is inconvenient and time consuming for a subject to respond, lower response rates should be expected. Although analytic conclusions are unreliable when response rates dip below 50%, analysis of data retrieved from response rates lower than 25% is not uncommon in the research literature. A key point to evaluate when assessing the adequacy of the sampling plan is not *how many* actually responded but *what percentage* responded. Even small samples may have good validity if they represent high response rates, and the reverse is also true—very large samples may hold little validity if they represent only a small fraction of the population.

Although there is no power calculation specifically for survey research, a general rule is that 15 responses should be solicited for every variable that is to be measured with the survey, exclusive of demographic descriptors. This number should be increased when subgroup analysis is planned. This means that larger samples will be needed for lengthy or complicated surveys or for studies in which differences between respondents will be analyzed based on some characteristic. The sample will need to be increased for expected nonrespondents. The usual practice is to survey at least twice as many subjects as you believe you need in the final sample.

Designing a Survey Research Study

Several systematic stages exist in the design of a survey research study. The first consideration is to define clearly the research question and the target population. As with any research question, it is worthwhile to consider these elements carefully, as they will drive many decisions that follow.

After it has been determined that the question is best answered by surveying a specific population, then the researcher develops a set of guiding questions or objectives that outline exactly what the researcher is trying to find out. At this point, outline any demographic characteristics that are of interest as well. This may take the form of a series of questions, a set of objectives, or a general outline.

The next step is to determine that no available instrument exists that is appropriate for the majority of the objectives. The word *majority* is impor-

---

Strengthen Your Survey Designs

Survey designs are some of the most common in health care and can help the bedside scientist incorporate the patient's preferences into the plan of care. Although they are common, they are not easily accomplished well. To assure you get the best possible evidence from a survey, try the following:

- Define the population carefully, and focus your definition to the smallest relevant group. With survey designs, the response *percentage* is more important than overall response numbers. With a large, poorly defined population, a 50% response rate is almost impossible to get.
- Keep the survey short and simple. Check the reading level, and get it down to no more than a sixth-grade level. Take out medical words, jargon, and acronyms. Measure only one concept with each question.
- Use instruments and surveys that have already been developed and tested for reliability and validity, even if they are not exactly what you need. It is better to revise an existing tool than to write one from scratch and test it yourself.
- Write a standardized protocol for administration of the tool, and use it consistently. Minimize measurement error by assuring the same directions are given each time the questionnaire is administered.
- Do not overgeneralize the results. Survey methods result in descriptive— or at best, correlation—data, and thus, we cannot quantify the effects of chance.

tant, as no survey will exactly measure what you need. However, it is worth using an instrument that is "close," or even revising one for your purposes, as developing an instrument from scratch is an arduous and time-consuming process. Testing for reliability and evaluating validity are all avoided when an existing instrument is available that has been tested for its psychometric properties.

If an instrument is located, its properties can be investigated using reports from the *Mental Measurements Yearbook*. Available for several decades, the *Mental Measurements Yearbook* allows for searches of available instruments and provides reviews of their usefulness in research. The *Mental Measurements Yearbook* can be accessed at most college or university libraries or via the web for a small fee.

If no instrument is located, then the researcher will need to develop one. The steps in instrument development include the following:

1. Write a series of questions that addresses each behavior, knowledge, skill, or attitude reflected in the objectives. In general, more questions are written than will eventually be needed so that they can be evaluated, changed, and removed if necessary.

2. Group the questions to reflect each major topic of the survey. Organize the questions from general (such as demographic characteristics) to specific. Format the survey so that is easy to follow and directions are uncomplicated.

3. Distribute a preliminary draft of the instrument to a group of colleagues who can review the document and identify problems with questions, including the way they are worded and the directions. Provide the group with copies of the objectives so they can determine if the questions will reasonably address each.

4. Revise the questionnaire, and test it on a pilot group of subjects. Measure the reliability of the instrument, and make any changes based on the statistical analysis or the feedback of the pilot group. (These subjects cannot be later included in the actual study or they will introduce the pretesting effect. Thus, keep this group small; 10 to 15 are sufficient.)

5. Analyze the results of the pilot group, looking for patterns of missing answers or inconsistency in responses, and make final revisions. Record the amount of time the subjects take to complete the survey.

An example of a survey appears in Appendix 2. This survey—used for a multidisciplinary bedside science project—had good reliability (alpha = 0.80) and demonstrates a range of question types.

Writing Good Survey Questions

Good survey questions are written using clear, uncomplicated language and simple instructions. Limit each question to a single concept to simplify both responses and analysis. Open-ended questions are useful for probing respondent's feelings. They have a lower response rate, however, and may be difficult to analyze.

Table 10-1   Examples of Survey Questions by Type

Type of Question	What It Is	Notes	An Example
Forced Choice	Questions that require the respondent to select from a predetermined list of answers	Forced choice questions are commonly used to describe the respondents or to measure their knowledge or recall. These are easy to analyze but do not allow for finding out information that is patient driven.	Which of the following aspects of the diabetic patient education program did you find most helpful? A. One-on-one contact with a nurse B. Group support with other diabetics C. Written materials for reference D. Web-based materials for reference
Dichotomous Choices	Questions that require the respondent to select from only two choices	Dichotomous questions measure the presence or absence of a given characteristic. These kinds of questions have limited analytic options, and it is difficult to measure reliability on dichotomous questions.	Are you presently involved in a diabetic patient education program? A. Yes B. No

Forced-choice questions require a response from a preselected list of possible responses. Scales may also be used, asking the respondent to rate each statement from "strongly disagree" to "strongly agree" or using some other standard for ranking. Forced-choice and scale questions are easier to analyze using quantitative methods but limit the responses available to the subject. Because these questions do not allow respondents to express their own personal viewpoints, they may produce biased data.

Table 10-1   Examples of Survey Questions by Type *(continued)*

Type of Question	What It Is	Notes	An Example
Scales	Questions that require the respondent to rank order their response on a continuum	Often referred to as Likert scales (after their original developer), scales are used to measure attitudes, perceptions, and beliefs.	How important do you believe it is to participate in a support group with other diabetics? A. Very important B. Important C. Somewhat important D. Not important
Open-Ended	Questions that ask for a free-form response from the respondent	Open-ended questions are useful for probing respondents' attitudes, beliefs, and opinions, without imposed limits. These questions can generate rich data but are difficult to analyze and must be treated as anecdotal and thus are not generalizable.	How could the diabetic patient education program be improved?

Data Collection Methods

Regardless of the design of the survey research, there is a singular focus for the data collection process: high-quality data that are reliable and valid. Many ways are available to collect survey information, and the choice of a data collection strategy depends on the nature of the research question, the specific information that is being gathered, and the resources available to the researcher.

Surveys may be administered with an interview. Interview surveys require the researcher to ask subjects specific questions and record their answers for later analysis. They may be done face-to-face or over the telephone. The latter has a lower response rate. To improve chances of success, solicit volunteers who are willing to give information over the telephone and schedule a specific data collection time at their convenience. Interviews are very labor intensive and, as a result, usually have small samples.

Questionnaires are also common survey data collection tools. Questionnaires are structured surveys that are self-administered by subjects. Questionnaires allow access to samples dispersed over large geographic areas if distributed through the mail or via the Internet. The associated anonymity encourages open and honest responses and reduces the effects of researcher bias. The standardized questions that are typical of questionnaires are identical for all subjects and thus result in more consistency of responses. These types of survey tools allow for quantitative analysis of responses and reliability of the instrument. Questionnaires suffer from the drawbacks of self-collected data, in that sampling error is introduced with this all-volunteer sample. In addition, response rate may suffer if the instrument is long or complicated.

Although paper-and-pencil surveys were the norm for many years—and still are the most common survey data collection method—web-based surveys are gaining popularity for several reasons. Web-based surveys are convenient for the subject because they can complete them at times and locations that are easiest for them. Surveys on the web are less costly for the researcher; no postage, envelopes, printing, or copying is required. Web-based surveys are more efficient for the researcher, as most survey software includes automatic reports that can be generated from the results, even while the study is in progress. It may be difficult, however, to get reliable e-mail addresses for large groups of subjects, and this inclusion criterion alone may result in a skewed sample, as the sample will be heavily weighted to those who are computer literate.

Analytic Procedures

Surveys are analyzed using primarily descriptive techniques. Demographic variables can be summarized using measures of central tendency (mean, median, standard deviation) or frequency tables based on the level of measure-

From the Mouths of Bedside Scientists: How Clinicians Talk About Survey Research

Why is it important to return surveys?

I never realized how important it was to return a survey until I did my own survey study about safety. We did a 40% random sample, but got only 20% of our surveys back. We looked at the results, but it was tough to make any decisions based on those results. Later, we redid the study and added incentives for responders. We got a much higher response rate, and we could much more confidently use our results. Now I am good about returning surveys because I have some empathy for the researcher.

What are some issues to be aware of when developing or using surveys?

I always thought I could pick and choose questions from an existing survey. It turns out, you cannot do that. All of the questions have to be taken together to be valid. I learned my lesson because I was told that I would have to revalidate a new survey I created. When I found out what was involved and how much time it would take, I decided to go with an existing, validated survey. Developing a survey is research in itself and is no little task.

I thought that if a survey was published, it would automatically be good. I found out the hard way. When I was presenting my research at a conference, a member of the audience made the comment that the survey tool that I used was not validated. That pretty much meant that my results were not necessarily true. Next time I will be sure to look up the research on the survey itself before I use it.

The way you write a question is very important. I probably did not fully understand this until some colleagues and I began developing a survey. We learned that you have to be very "unambiguous" and that it is important to have someone outside of the group read and comment on your questions. We also found out the order of questions can be important. When we piloted our survey with patients, we found out that we were not even asking the right questions to address our problem. Because this was a stroke patient population, we realized that instead of asking the patient who often could not respond well, we should have been talking to a family member. Next time, we plan to start with a focus group of the patients we plan to study. Survey research is truly a challenging science in itself.

ment. These data are often best presented in tables or graphs. If there are more than 200 subjects in the response set, then even scaled data can be summarized with measures of central tendency. If there are fewer than 200, then frequency tables should be used for analysis.

Often, researchers are interested in whether two or more answers are related or whether certain answers are related to demographic characteristics. The most common analytic technique for these questions is the correlation coefficient.

At its most fundamental, survey research is descriptive. Although correlations between responses may be described, surveys are not commonly used for inference. As a result, statistics that reflect the probability of sampling error (reported as p values) are not relevant and are rarely used in reporting survey results.

QUALITATIVE RESEARCH

Qualitative research is an exploratory research method that is used to study phenomena when quantitative methods are not appropriate and survey methods are too restrictive. Qualitative studies investigate attitudes, feelings, and beliefs of respondents through naturalistic inquiry, noninterfering data collection techniques, and a concern for context. The goal of qualitative research is to depict an experience in such depth that one who has not experienced it can understand it. Qualitative research is an emergent design, with few prior constraints regarding methods or analysis. Some specific procedures, however, do help assure that validity is maximized and bias is minimized so that conclusions are accurate.

Sampling Strategies

Qualitative research has a goal of understanding meaning, not producing generalizable knowledge. The rules for probability sampling, central to experimental designs, are not relevant for qualitative studies. The goal is to capture the words of informants so that meaning can be determined, and this requires subjects that are rich in information and willing to share their experiences. A deliberate and purposeful approach for subject selection is the norm rather than an objective and random one.

The specific sampling strategy is driven by the research question, the type of study, the breadth of information needed, and the general purpose of the research. The researcher should carefully consider each of these and report a rationale for the sampling strategy. Basically, respondents are selected because they can best inform the research question, however, and any other considerations are secondary in qualitative research.

The subjects for a qualitative study are selected based on a general set of inclusion criteria but otherwise are often samples of convenience and accessibility. As with experimental designs, a qualitative study should report sample inclusion criteria, recruiting methods, and attrition. Descriptive statistics about the sample, such as the distribution of age, gender, and other relevant characteristics, should be provided. These may be the only numbers reported in the entire study.

The sample must be sufficient to achieve depth of understanding, but sample sizes may be quite small. Instead of judging samples by their power, a different standard is used to determine when a sufficient sample size has been achieved. This state—called saturation—is determined by the researcher when it is concluded that no new information is being generated. This is clearly a subjective judgment, but one that is made impartially and based on the evidence that has been produced. Samples may be as small as a single subject that is studied in a great deal of depth or may involve many more individuals through focus groups or observation. There are no preset rules for sample size in qualitative studies other than the standard of determining that saturation has been met before concluding data collection.

Types of Qualitative Designs

There are many qualitative designs, but a relative few are appropriate for evidence-based practice studies. Those that answer clinical questions best are as follows:

Content analysis: In this most common qualitative study, individuals or focus groups are interviewed to determine their thoughts, beliefs, attitudes, or perceptions related to a specific research question. Content analysis is usually based on analysis of spoken words but may involve print materials or observation as well. Content analysis might be used to determine how patients feel about restricted visiting in critical care areas, and how visiting policies could be changed to better meet the needs of patients and their families.

Case study: The study of a single case in depth over time is a common qualitative design in health studies, particularly when studying rare conditions. A "case" may be a person, an event, a program, a time period, or even an entire patient care unit. The case study provides a richly detailed portrait to provide in-depth understanding of the characteristics and responses of the individual under study. An example of a case study might be the observation of how the parents of a chronically ill child interact with the caregivers.

Ethnography: Ethnography is the study of an entire group of people to understand their culture. Ethnography is usually accomplished with mixed methods, including observation, interaction, and interview. An example of an ethnography might be the study of the effects of culture on the behavior of families in waiting rooms.

Phenomenology: Phenomenology is the study of groups of individuals that share the same experience or characteristic. An example of a phenomenological study might be the investigation of the coping strategies used by women who have diagnosed breast cancer.

Control of Internal Validity

Internal validity is less of an issue in qualitative research. After all, the fundamental meaning of internal validity is that the effect of an intervention can be isolated from all other effects. Because qualitative research makes no

---

Strengthen Your Qualitative Designs

Qualitative research is difficult and time consuming to do. Limit its use to important questions that cannot be answered in any other way. You will do best collecting qualitative data if you:

- Limit data collection to only one or two key questions. Trying to gather too much data will bog down data analysis and make it difficult to draw valid conclusions.
- Talk through your biases with a neutral party before starting the study. This method of "bracketing" your bias helps you put them aside by recognizing what they are.
- Choose the subjects carefully. Subjects should be those who can best inform the question, even if they are selected purposefully. Setting specific inclusion and exclusion criteria can reduce selection effects.
- Use the standard of saturation to determine sample size. When you say to yourself, "I'm not hearing anything new here," then it's likely saturation has been reached.
- Keep a log of decisions that you make about the study. These serve as an audit trail and can be a learning tool for your future qualitative efforts.
- Try to get multiple sources of information (e.g., patient satisfaction data as well as interviews). This represents efforts to triangulate data and enhances internal validity.

claims of linking causes to their effects and is a fundamentally descriptive study, isolating alternative explanations is not relevant. That is not to say that there are not some steps a qualitative researcher can do to control *bias*, the major threat to internal validity in any type of study.

In experimental research, the primary sources of bias are the researcher, the measurement, and the subjects. In qualitative research, the researcher *is* the measurement instrument. The researcher and the subjects, then, are the primary sources of bias.

The primary methods used to control internal validity in qualitative studies are those aimed at controlling bias relative to the researcher and the subjects. Researchers use *bracketing* as a method of recognizing and setting aside their opinions about a study. By requiring themselves to specifically identify biases, the reader can take into account the potential role of researcher bias in the outcome. A researcher can strengthen validity by producing an *audit trail*. An audit trail, sometimes called a *decision trail*, is a detailed description of each decision that emerged during design and data collection. Although not intended to guide replication of the study, it does enable the reader to evaluate the effects of design decisions on validity. *Triangulation* is a strong control for internal validity. Triangulation is the use of three or more independent sources to verify a conclusion from qualitative data.

Although these methods do not assure the control of researcher bias, they help the reader to have more confidence in the findings of the researchers because they make the research processes more transparent. Other threats to validity are *selection effects*, or bias created by the way the sample is selected, and *treatment effects*, which are artificial responses from the subjects. Subjects may also be unable to recall, be dishonest, or misunderstand questions. Some of these *subject effects* can be mitigated by the strategy of *member checking*, in which the conclusions of the researchers are reviewed and validated by the subjects. This final step— of presenting results to respondents and making adjustments—is a key method for increasing both the dependability and credibility of the researcher's findings.

Each of these controls for internal validity enhances a different aspect of the qualitative study and thus use of more than one control method is desirable. The strongest qualitative evidence will come from research studies that use all or most of these common methods to enhance internal validity.

Data Collection Methods

Qualitative data may be collected using a variety of methods. Many studies use more than one data collection method, enhancing validity through triangu-

Hitting the Stacks

Qualitative research is characterized by purposive sampling or samples that are selected explicitly because they can best inform the research question. This does not mean samples are selected subjectively; sampling criteria should be developed to guide the selection of subjects. Mactavish and Iwasaki (2005) used this approach in their study of stress-coping among people with disabilities: "A criterion-based purposive sampling technique was used to identify prospective participants from this pool. The selection criteria required that (a) the individual have a diagnosed form of disability, preferably one that resulted in permanent mobility impairment, and (b) relatively equal representation of people by sex and age."

The nature of purposive sampling means it will be descriptive and will not be generalizable. A reasonable goal, however, is to transfer the results to like subjects and settings. This limited external validity can still be compromised by various threats, as these researchers found when historical events interfered with attaining a gender-balanced sample. "Generally, it was more challenging to recruit male participants, and of the eight who confirmed their willingness . . . only half actually attended. . . . This low rate was likely exacerbated by severe weather (snow storm) on the day of the session."

The analytic procedure and controls for validity should be equally transparent. Iaquinta and Larrabee (2004) conducted a phenomenological study of the experience of patients living with rheumatoid arthritis. Their thorough description of the coding process, as well as the steps taken to control bias (bracketing, thick description, member checking), strengthen the validity of their findings: "First, the descriptive accounts were read to determine the overall sense of meaning. The next step involved rereading the descriptive accounts, extracting the significant statements (150), and eliminating redundancy. The researcher bracketed presuppositions, biases, and personal influences during the analysis. The third step identified formulating meanings imbedded in the significant statements. Then, six clusters of themes emerged from the formulated meanings. There was no reflection or intentional recall of information from the review of literature completed at the beginning of the research study. The fifth step resulted in a rich, exhaustive description of the phenomena. Validation was secured by the participants' confirmation of the findings, and no relevant data emerged."

Mactavish, J., & Y. Iwasaki. 2005. Exploring perspectives of individuals with disabilities on stress-coping. *Journal of Rehabilitation* 71: 20–31.

Iaquinta, M., & J. Larrabee. 2004. Phenomenological lived experience of patients with rheumatoid arthritis. *Journal of Nursing Care Quality* 19: 280–89.

lation. All of the methods have in common a focus on describing, in words, an experience or observation. This may take the form of any or all of these:

- *Interview*: Data are collected directly from subjects by one-on-one interviews with the researcher. An interview guide may or may not be used. A hallmark of qualitative interviews is the open-ended question. In general, only a few questions are used and the subjects guide where the interview goes. This method yields rich data but requires a great deal of time and effort on the part of both the researcher and the subject and requires that the researcher have capable interviewing skills.
- *Focus groups*: Multiple subjects can provide data simultaneously via a focus group. Focus groups are groups of individuals that share some common experience or characteristic for a facilitated discussion. Usually no more than 8 to 10 people participate, and the researcher generally asks open-ended questions using an unstructured interview guide. Focus groups have the advantage of providing data from multiple subjects in a time-effective way, but they, too, require a skilled facilitator and motivated subjects.
- *Observation*: Qualitative data may be gathered directly by the researcher through extended observation and detailed descriptions. Called *thick description*, observations are recorded in minute detail over an extended period of time to determine patterns of responses or general behavioral themes.

All data collection procedures result in the same thing—a large amount of data recorded as descriptive phrases, words, and the quotes of subjects. Although the raw data at this point are only a compilation of anecdotes, analytic processes are systematic and rigorous to assure that conclusions are based on patterns and themes in the data and can be confirmed with analytic methods.

Analytic Procedures

Qualitative data are words rather than numbers. As such, they are analyzed by interpretation rather than mathematical manipulation. Instead of calculating statistical significance and probability, meaning is extracted from the words. The researcher still needs to use thoughtful care when drawing conclusions from the data. A systematic process should be used and described thoroughly so that the reader can follow how the conclusions were reached.

Because the data are words and not numbers, the tables and graphs that are common in experimental studies are missing. Instead, the researcher should report the words of informants as supporting "data" for their conclusions. This use of the verbatim words of those in the study adds validity to the conclusions, as the reader can draw his or her own conclusions as to whether the themes that are identified by the author seem supported by the subjects' words.

Qualitative data may be analyzed using a variety of methods, but the most common is content analysis. The verbatim transcripts and notes are reviewed for tone, and phrases are aggregated to determine general themes. Each level of analysis is increasingly detailed, until overarching themes are supported by more detailed descriptions of patterns in the data, called codes. The validity of conclusions can be strengthened by having two raters code the data and measuring their level of agreement, called interrater reliability. Common statistics that might be reported for interrater reliability include chi square, Cohen's kappa, and the correlation coefficient. In any case, interrater agreement of greater than 85% is desirable.

The researcher should report the specific process used for analysis, the final themes (there should not be very many) and supporting codes for the

For more depth and detail, try these resources:

Aday, L.A. 1996. *Designing and Conducting Health Surveys,* 2nd ed. San Francisco: Jossey Bass.

Biswanathan, M. 2005. *Measurement Error and Research Design.* Thousand Oaks, CA: Sage Publications.

Crawford, C., S. McCabe, and D. Pope. 2005. Applying web-based survey design standards. *Journal of Prevention & Intervention in the Community* 29: 43–66.

Denzin, N.K., and Y.S. Lincoln. 2000. *Handbook of Qualitative Research,* 2nd ed. Thousand Oaks, CA: Sage Publications.

Johnson, R., & J. Waterfield. 2004. Making words count: The value of qualitative research. *Physiotherapy Research International* 9: 121–131.

Krueger, R., and M. Casey. 2000. *Focus Groups: A Practical Guide for Applied Research.* Thousand Oaks, CA: Sage Publications.

Nardi, P. 2002. *Doing Survey Research: A Guide to Quantitative Research Methods.* Boston: Allyn and Bacon.

Neuendorf, K.A. 2002. *The Content Analysis Guidebook.* Thousand Oaks, CA: Sage Publications.

Sandelowski, M. 2004. Using qualitative research. *Qualitative Health Research* 14: 1366–86.

Yin, R.K. 2003. *Case Study Research: Design and Methods,* 3rd ed. Thousand Oaks, CA: Sage Publications.

themes. Quotes from subjects should confirm each code, serving as supporting evidence.

USING THE RESULTS

Although survey and qualitative data are rated low for use in evidence-based practice, their results can still provide valuable insights into why clinical practices may or may not work. Patients' and staff feelings and perceptions can affect the way they interact with each other and adhere to the plan of care. In addition, some clinical considerations are not easily observed—such as pain, or nausea, or depression—and are best measured by asking respondents directly.

The best survey studies for application to clinical practice are those that have been carried out on a clearly defined population, using sound sampling strategies and reliable measurement techniques. These studies have the broadest application to clinical practice and use in patient care.

Qualitative research is not intended for generalizability. That does not mean the results cannot be transferred to other similar situations and patients. In the case of both survey and qualitative studies—as with any study—a careful consideration of the nature of the subjects, the setting, and the methods will help you determine whether the results can be reasonably applied to your situation.

SUMMARY

Survey and qualitative designs can be effective research methods for gathering information directly from respondents about their attitudes, perceptions, feelings, or beliefs. Both designs are best done with a systematic approach and attention to design principles. Samples for surveys should be large and randomly selected for best generalizability. Effort should be made to find or develop instruments that measure the questions of the study with reliability and validity.

Qualitative studies have purposefully selected samples and open-ended data collection techniques. Analysis is accomplished by finding patterns or themes in the data. Several methods can help control internal validity of qualitative studies, including researcher bias bracketing, triangulation, development of an audit trail, member checking, and careful sampling strategies.

Survey and qualitative data are best used to fill gaps in clinical knowledge that relate to attitudes, beliefs, and values. These studies can help us consider patient preferences when designing best practice guidelines.

Concepts in Action

Survey research can have qualitative and quantitative aspects; clinically important information can be obtained from both. Familiarity with qualitative and survey methods can be very helpful to bedside scientists when they are exploring a topic. These methods can be used to capture information that cannot be obtained with quantitative methods. Understanding attitudes, perceptions, motives, and psychosocial aspects of care often requires survey and qualitative methods. These methods are good for answering *why* and *how* questions. It is very common that quantitative and qualitative data collection methods are used together in the same study. As you read the following study, you will notice how it illustrates aspects of both qualitative and survey research using this "mixed method" approach.

What were the questions studied in this bedside science project?
What factors are perceived as affecting satisfaction by patients and their families in the waiting room environment of a level I trauma center's emergency department?

Why was this research question important?
Patient and family satisfaction is considered an important aspect of a patient's healthcare experience. Because the emergency department is often an individual's first exposure to a hospital facility, what happens in the waiting room can have a powerful influence on the entire hospital care experience.

Who was involved on the research team?
The team was collaborative in that it included nurse administrators, medical staff, a patient representative, an analyst, and healthcare research specialists. Also important to this team was the input of a medical anthropologist, who provided expertise in qualitative research methods. The medical anthropologist shared experiences from other studies that evaluated intensive care unit waiting room experiences.

What methods were planned?
The team developed a research plan based on patient admission rates and research resources. They chose a mixed methods approach, using qualitative and quantitative methods of evaluation. Both scientific literature and internal data were used for analysis. The team also planned for systematic observation of the waiting room, mapped patient flow on a scaled map of the waiting room, and designed an emergency department waiting room satisfaction survey.

Concepts in Action *(continued)*

Evaluation of Waiting Room Structure

The team started with an evaluation of the structure of the waiting room. A detailed description of the layout and contents of the room was developed. Photographs were taken of all sections of the waiting room to evaluate lighting, décor, and furniture layout. This area was mapped and patient type (adult, child, handicapped in wheelchair, etc.) was recorded. The primary aim of this part of the study was to evaluate any potential issues related to seating arrangements and room layout.

Survey Development

Because no acceptable surveys were found in the literature that specifically evaluated satisfaction with the emergency room waiting room environment, the team decided that their first task would be to develop a survey. A draft questionnaire was developed based on prior patient complaints and the specific research questions of team members. The team was fortunate to have a copy of the questionnaire created for the intensive care unit waiting room study as a basis for their work. To protect patient identity and encourage honest answers, the team decided on an anonymous survey that would be dropped in a locked box.

The draft questionnaire was then pilot tested with a small group of patients and their families (n = 38). Nurses and other emergency department staff were asked to evaluate and rate the appropriateness of each question and to suggest additional questions. Pilot questionnaire data were then reviewed, and the questionnaire was refined. The final survey had 14 Likert-type questions and seven open-ended questions. Topics covered by the survey were the waiting room environment, telephones, staff presence and behavior, traffic, availability of food, triage processes, child-specific issues, privacy, and parking. Minimal demographics were asked to maintain confidentiality. The patient's Emergency Severity Index (ESI) was written on the top of the questionnaire before it was handed to the patient. The ESI is a measure of the patient's severity that defines unique aspects of emergency department processes of care, and the team felt it was an important demographic that they might want to explore further during the analysis phase.

Simple face and content validity of the questionnaire were established using experienced emergency department nurse leaders. The final questionnaire was distributed over a 2-week period, at random times on random days, in a way that captured time-based differences.

(continues)

Concepts in Action (continued)

Questionnaire Process

The triage nurse wrote the patient's ESI scores on the questionnaire and gave it to the patient after the initial intake session, with instructions for him or her or a family member to complete the survey while he or she was in the waiting room. Patients and families were assured that all comments were strictly confidential and were to be placed in a locked box at the volunteer's desk. Nurses made a tick mark on a flow sheet for each survey distributed. A total of 53 surveys were returned, for a calculated 82% return rate.

Emergency Department Waiting Room Observations

As a group, the team chose a 3-week observation period to coincide with the distribution of the surveys. Six team members were trained to do observations. Observers used a narrative format to document detailed descriptions of what they saw and heard in the waiting room environment at random times and during random days. They used a scaled map of the waiting room and its furniture to document location of individuals and objects (e.g., wheelchairs). They recorded the number of individuals in the waiting room, along with the date and time of day at the beginning and end of each observation.

Evaluating the Data

Observation narratives and open-ended responses were typed from the hand-written forms to electronic files and then themed (i.e., a topic area was assigned to groups of information). The themed data were grouped by day of week, then time of day, and then by ESI score to evaluate trends. Demographic data were reported as frequencies, and Likert-scale data were reported as box plots. There was a good distribution of respondents across all age groups. ESI scores of the subjects were proportional to the usual distribution of patient severity scores, and thus, the ability to generalize to the larger population was strengthened.

When responses were grouped by ESI score, the team noticed what appeared to be differences in survey scores by severity group. This suspicion was confirmed with a Mann Whitney U test for nonparametric data (because these data were from scales) that showed statistically significant differences between severity groups.

What challenges were faced?

The team was frustrated because the number of family and/or patients in the waiting room was dramatically lower than expected. During the

Concepts in Action *(continued)*

study, the number of individuals in the waiting room ranged from 0 to 18, and frequently, there were no more than 8 people present. Projections were that 20 to 30 individuals would be present at any given time, based on numbers reported in earlier studies. Wait times were also much lower than expected, with most waits less than 1 hour, and frequently only 5 to 15 minutes passed from arrival to treatment. Earlier studies documented waits of more than an hour, and the shorter wait times in this study may have affected results.

Many other improvement projects were also in progress, and issues arose related to sharing of data and project resources. These issues were addressed through ongoing communication efforts throughout the study and as study results were reported.

How was this study used?

Information from this baseline study was used to make changes that addressed the concerns of patients and families about the waiting room environment. Some changes were relatively easy to implement and were immediately put in place, including the following:

- A more visible presence of security personnel
- Replacing the old phone books
- Assuring cleanliness of the bathrooms
- Reminding staff of the obligation to patient confidentiality
- Reinforcement of the qualities expected of volunteers who welcomed patients and checked on their well-being
- Updating reading materials

Other changes took longer, including a playhouse to give children a safe place to play, new chairs, and better furniture layout. Changes planned in the long term include investigation of cell phone technology and improved access for family members.

How were results communicated internally and to larger audiences?

Information from this project was shared with staff from the emergency department during the staff meeting. This team presented the results as an oral presentation at the hospital's research day and as a symposium presentation at a national conference. This team is in the process of publishing their study methods and baseline results.

Checklist for Evaluating a Survey Study

_____ The survey method is appropriate for the research question.

_____ The population is clearly defined.

_____ The sample is selected randomly and represents the given population.

_____ Response rate is greater than 50%, irrespective of actual numbers of responses.

_____ At least 15 subjects responded for each variable measured.

_____ Instruments are documented as reliable and valid (as appropriate).

_____ Interviewers are trained in interviewing techniques (as appropriate).

_____ Results are analyzed using appropriate descriptive statistics and measures of correlation.

Checklist for Evaluating a Qualitative Research Study

_____ The design is easily determined and linked to the research question.

_____ Inclusion criteria, recruiting method, and demographic characteristics of the sample are reported.

_____ Saturation is reported and used as a method of determining final sample size.

_____ Bracketing is used to control the impact of researcher bias.

_____ Data conclusions are confirmed by at least three separate sources of data (triangulation).

_____ A clear audit trail describes each design decision and is detailed enough for replication.

_____ Conclusions and themes are confirmed by member checking.

_____ Interrater reliability is tested and reported to confirm dependability of coding.

CHAPTER 11

Communicating Your Findings: The Final Step

In this chapter, you will learn to

- Select the right target audience for your research
- Prepare an abstract for submission to a conference or journal editor
- Develop a compelling poster presentation
- Prepare and comfortably deliver a podium presentation
- Submit a manuscript for publication in a peer-reviewed journal

After much hard work, your study is complete, and you are proud of the findings. You learned a great deal about the realities of conducting research in a bedside setting, and your study dispelled some myths about costly and—as it turned out—ineffective treatments. Your family and friends are tired of hearing about the study; thus, it is time to reach a larger audience, one that can use your findings. Where should you start? The study is well done; you controlled most extraneous variables, had a strong sampling strategy, and used good measures and analyses. It might be good enough for publication, but you decide to start by getting your research peer reviewed. You find a "call for posters" from a professional association's annual conference and send off an abstract.

After 2 months, when you have nearly forgotten your submission, you get a notice in the mail: Your poster has been accepted at the conference. This is exciting! You seek help from your research department in deciding what should go on the poster, and your media center helps to prepare the poster. At the conference, there is considerable interest in your research, and more than two dozen individuals approach you and ask for more detail about the study. The encouragement you receive is gratifying, and you are surprised at how satisfying it is to have your hard work recognized.

Knowing that your peers have reviewed the study and found it acceptable, you submit an abstract for a podium presentation at a conference. Success again! You have been asked to present a 30-minute research presentation to your professional colleagues at the conference. Although nervous, you are thoroughly prepared, and your presentation is well received. You surprise even yourself with your comfortable and relaxed responses to questions and realize that, on this specific topic at least, you are the expert. After the presentation, a journal editor encourages you to submit the research for publication. Your excitement over this feedback is tempered by your reluctance—you have never written professionally before and have not put together a research report since you were in college. Where should you start? What should you include? How can you make sure the article is interesting and easy to read? You want to make sure you take advantage of this opportunity to share what you have found and showcase your efforts.

Communicating the results of research cannot stop with organizational changes in policies and procedures. Part of the purpose of research of any kind—practice based or otherwise—is to make a contribution to the body of empirical knowledge that is the foundation of a profession. There are many ways to communicate research so that it can be incorporated into practice— local, regional, and national conferences often solicit both poster and podium presentations, and journals are always receptive to solid research studies on relevant clinical topics. In contrast to what many clinicians may think, journals are often anxious to publish works by staff level practitioners, as those closest to clinical processes are often in the best position to determine how to improve them.

Inexperienced researchers may feel that their work is not sophisticated or important enough for publication or presentation. In reality, good work is good work, regardless of who conducts it. The process of getting a research study reviewed is systematic and one that is available to any researcher, whether seasoned or novice. A common approach for a new researcher is to follow the steps of submitting research for peer review as a poster in a regional or national conference, followed by podium presentations and, finally, publication in a peer-reviewed publication. Regardless of the venue chosen for peer review, the basic steps are the same.

SELECT THE RIGHT AUDIENCE

The first step in communicating the findings of a research study is to select the right audience for your work. Consider the target audience before writing the abstract or preparing the manuscript. The best venue is one that has a clearly defined focus that fits your work. Some are clear—a study on reducing infections would obviously be appropriate for conferences and journals that focus on infection control—but others are not. Look for journal titles that "fit" with your study. Some journals publish lists of priorities or solicitations for articles on their web pages or in the journal itself. Conferences generally include a list of conference objectives or goal statements that cover the types of information that are of interest. The more closely you can match the study topic with a topic of interest for the journal or conference, the more likely that you will be successful with your submissions.

The best audience is one that can put your results into practice. Select a conference or periodical that will provide access to the clinicians who are in the best position to apply what you have found. After you have picked an appropriate audience—whether for a conference or a journal—prepare a compelling abstract of your work that best gets across what you have accomplished.

PREPARE A CONCISE ABSTRACT (AND FOLLOW THE RULES)

After you have identified the appropriate location for your submission, read the instructions for authors carefully. Conferences have very specific requirements for submissions, including spacing, margins, and method of submissions. Pay particular attention to limits on the number of words and deadlines. Personnel who screen submissions for reviewers often discard abstracts that violate the fundamental instructions, and thus, your abstract may not even reach reviewers if it is too long or in the wrong format. Submissions after the deadline are generally not reviewed at all; thus, be sure to submit your abstract by the date noted in the conference materials.

The abstract of your work is the only description that most conference reviewers will see, and it may be the first description that a journal editor sees. It should be clear, compelling, and concise. The abstract should report the most important elements of your research in a way that generates interest and even excitement about your project. Think of the abstract as an advertisement for your research, focusing on the strongest points and most interesting findings.

Check the conference or journal specifics for the length of the abstract. Some limit the abstract to as little as 100 words—others allow up to 500. Take care not to exceed the word length. If the conference or journal provides direction as to what must be included in the abstract, follow its guidance carefully. It helps to put each required element as a heading in bold font so that the reviewer can find the various sections easily and determine that all are present without having to read the abstract multiple times. Many times no specific guidelines are provided. In this case, use the generally accepted standards for what is included in an abstract; they appear in Table 11-1.

Table 11-1   Anatomy of a Research Abstract

Element	What Is Included
Introduction	Usually use no more than a sentence or two. Answer this question: Why is this research important? Include provocative sentences or an interesting lead in that will "grab" the reader so that he or she will want to read the entire abstract. Do not use extraneous information, jokes, or clichés; you do not have the luxury of using words for information that are not central to the research. This section may be called "Introduction," "Summary," or "Background."
Objective	Report the primary purpose of the study; this can be one or two sentences that describe the aim of the study in detail. If the research question is a restatement of the purpose statement, do not include both. If, on the other hand, the purpose is achieved with an unconventional research question, then include both. This section may be called "Objective," "Purpose," or "Aims."
Methods	Describe the design of the study, the methods used to achieve the purpose, and the procedures applied to control internal validity.

Write the abstract, and then edit multiple times until the word length is achieved. Focus on the most important information that communicates the study strengths and usefulness. Have another professional review the abstract and comment on its clarity, completeness, and the relevance of the information that has been included. When you have reviewed the abstract several times and are confident that it represents your study well, send it for peer review. Expect the peer review process to take from 2 weeks to several months; the guidelines for submission should give an indication of when you can expect a response from the reviewers. Do not assume that no an-

---

Table 11-1   **Anatomy of a Research Abstract** *(continued)*

Element	What Is Included
Methods *(continued)*	This should include the sampling strategy and the analytic plan. Identify the independent and dependent variables, which may also be called "predictors" and "outcomes." Enough detail should be presented that the reader understands the fundamental process for the research, but do not overload with detail. Only minimal statistics are included, but these usually include the sample size and the calculated power. The actual statistical tests that were run should be explicitly identified.
Results	Summarize the most important results (whether they were statistically significant or not). Keep in mind that a lack of effect may be as important as the presence of one. Some statistical results may be reported here but limit these to test statistics and associated p values. Do not use this section to comment on the meaning of the results, but simply report them.
Conclusions	Focus on the most important implications of the findings and the usefulness for practice. Application issues should be addressed here.

swer is a negative answer. It is acceptable to check on the status of your abstract if you have heard nothing in 4 to 6 weeks, especially if it is a large conference.

When your abstract is accepted, you will be notified if it is to be presented as a poster or a podium presentation. The work of preparing your research as a presentation then begins.

PREPARE A COMPELLING POSTER

A poster presentation at a conference is a research report presented as a visual display so that it can be read and viewed by large groups of professionals in an informal setting. The author stands near the poster at specified times to discuss the details of the research and answer questions. A poster presentation gives the author an opportunity to interact with participants and discuss their research. Poster presentations are a good place for a novice researcher to start the communication process because it is less intimidating than a podium presentation and requires less preparation than a formal manuscript. Nevertheless, abstracts for poster presentations are peer reviewed and accepted based on merit, and thus, they begin the scholarly review process that is the hallmark of professional research.

After an abstract has been accepted as a poster presentation, the process of poster development begins. Allow plenty of time for this process, as the elements of the poster must be decided on, developed, and translated into physical form. This requires the help of specialists in both research and media development; thus, allow sufficient time for others to make their contribution.

Check the specifications for the poster before beginning its development. Each conference will have specific requirements for the size of the poster, the length of time it can be displayed, and the amount of time you will be expected to be present. Take advantage of all of the space available for your poster, and plan to be present whenever you are allowed to maximize exposure and communication of your findings.

When you are clear on the limitations for your poster, begin by drawing a rough sketch of the poster first. The purpose of a poster is to translate ideas and images into graphic form, and thus, plan to *show* the viewer what you have done instead of telling them. It is helpful to develop a mockup of the poster using graph paper and sticky notes to get an idea of the layout that will be effective as well as how much space you will need for each element.

Although handouts are helpful and appreciated at conferences, the poster should serve as a stand-alone description of your research. Ask yourself what information is absolutely central to understanding your research and its clini-

Strengthen Your Poster Presentation

- A poster presentation is a visual medium; thus, try to *show* what was done instead of using text. Arrows, flowcharts, diagrams, photographs, and schematics may all be used to demonstrate your research instead of describing it.
- Use bullets in the text. These emphasis points make the material easier to follow and read, and add interest to the presentation.
- When in doubt, edit out. Cluttered posters are hard to read and may be disregarded. Make sure every item on the poster is necessary. The purpose is to stimulate discussion, not formally report every detail of the research.
- Use a neutral colored background for the poster. It is easier on the eyes than bright colors and will not distract from the information on the poster or clash with the colors in your charts. Use white space effectively to differentiate parts of the poster and accentuate the elements.
- Self-explanatory graphics should dominate the poster. Although you may be present to discuss your work in more detail, not every individual who looks at the poster will have an opportunity to discuss it with you. The work should stand alone as a general report of the research.
- Text and graphics should be readable from a distance of 4 to 6 feet. Sans serif fonts (fonts without embellishments) are easiest to read. Vary the font size relative to the importance of the information.
- The flow of the poster should be from left to right and top to bottom. Labeling each element with a number helps the reader sequence the parts of the poster in a logical way.

cal implications; begin with this content and expand on it as space allows. The usual components of a poster include the following:

- *Introduction*: The introduction attracts attention to the poster, summarizes the identified need for the research, and describes the significance of the study. Statistics reporting the prevalence of the clinical problem and the clinical implications are helpful.
- *Research purpose and question*: The purpose statement and research question help focus the study and identify the exact aim of the work.
- *Methods and design*: This section should include a concise description of the design, procedures, measures, and analytic tests used in the study.

- *Results:* Results should be presented in primarily visual form, using tables or graphs, with limited text.
- *Conclusions*: Although brief, the conclusions are the heart of the poster. This section should highlight the most significant findings and implications for clinicians.
- *Acknowledgments*: Include recognition of staff who helped with the research or the poster and the sponsors of the project. You should also note here whether any funding was received that supported the project.
- *References*: A brief reference list, focusing on the most important citations, can be included at the end of the poster.

Figure 11-1 represents the typical layout of a poster, with associated text font sizes and content. There are, however, infinite ways to lay out a poster so that it is readable and draws the viewer in to find out more. A poster can be an effective way to interact with those who are interested in the research and to present the study in an informal setting. Podium presentations, on the other hand, provide the opportunity to reach a large audience in a relatively short period of time while providing more information than is possible in a poster presentation.

PRESENTING YOUR RESEARCH EFFECTIVELY

The communication skills that are needed to present research effectively are not different from those needed for any type of group presentation—effective preparation, practice, and focused content development. To prepare for a podium presentation, you will need to know the type of talk that is expected, the composition of the audience, the amount of time you have, and the objectives for your presentation. Adequately understanding each of these can help you communicate your research in a way that maximizes dissemination of your findings while keeping your anxiety to a minimum.

What Type of Presentation Is Expected?

The types of research presentations can vary from an informal roundtable discussion to a highly formalized keynote speech. The kind of presentation will drive the content; thus, be clear on what is expected before you begin preparations. Different types of presentations have different objectives. If you are in doubt as to the goals for your presentation, ask for direction from your contact person. Specifically determine what audiovisual support to expect and whether projection equipment is available. It is not uncommon that a projector is provided but that the speaker is expected to bring a laptop computer; thus, verify what you will need to bring with you. Check on the portable media that will work, as well; do not assume that the computer will have a floppy

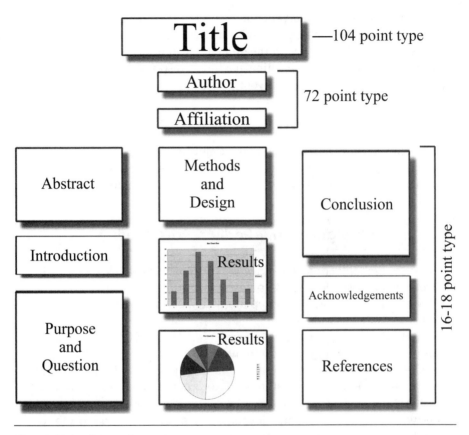

Figure 11-1   A sample poster.

drive ("A" drive) or compact disk reader. Ask the conference organizers for specifics. You will also want to know whether handouts will be made available or whether you will have to bring your own supplements with you.

Who Will Be the Audience for Your Presentation?

The composition of the audience will also drive the development of your presentation. Whether the audience is composed of generalists or specialists will dictate the level of detail you provide. The number of participants and where they come from is also important; an international audience needs a different presentation style than a domestic one. Their educational level and current knowledge of the material are also helpful to know, as you can tailor your presentation so that it is neither too complicated nor too simplified. It is also helpful to know how the audience may apply the information and whether they will focus on usefulness of the information rather than theoretical considerations. In-depth knowledge of the audience will help you to customize the presentation to their needs, resulting in a better response on the part of the attendees and less apprehension on your part.

How Much Time Do You Have?

Two considerations in managing the timeframe for your presentation are these: how much time you have to prepare materials, and how much time you have to present at the conference. Many conferences prepare reference books

Strengthen Your Podium Presentation

- Podium presentations often have very tight timeframes. When you develop your outline for the presentation, allocate a portion of the time allowed to each section. Develop the detail for each section with these time constraints in mind.
- Practice, practice, practice. Time yourself (there is a built-in timer in PowerPoint), and practice some more until you are well within the allotted time. A novice presenter is one who goes over the time limit. If you use slides, keep in mind that 2 to 3 minutes of talking time per slide is the average; do not overload your presentation.
- Have colleagues attend one of your practice sessions and provide you with a critique. Often, someone unfamiliar with your research can tell you where your presentation has gaps or is confusing. Ask for feedback about your presentation style as well as content so that you can gain confidence in both aspects.
- Using a presentation package such as PowerPoint can enhance your delivery—or detract from it. Although slides can help hold the attention of the audience, busy backgrounds or slides crowded with text can actually pull attention away from you. A basic rule is no more than seven lines to a slide and no more than seven words to a line. Stay away from light backgrounds—they are hard on the eyes when projected.
- If you have detailed statistics or tables, put them on a handout instead of a slide. Simple graphs are helpful, but too much detail cannot be read from a distance and distracts the audience.
- Speak naturally; pauses are a normal part of speech, as are gestures. Keep a professional stance, however, with your hands out of your pockets and your arms naturally relaxed.

for attendees that include summaries or notes from each presentation. The publication deadlines for these references are much earlier than the actual start date of the conference; thus, you may be asked to submit your handouts and other materials as much as 6 months before the conference. Check these deadlines carefully when you receive your acceptance materials so that you have plenty of time to prepare good supplemental materials.

The second time-related concern is the actual amount of time you have for the presentation. Be sure to subtract 5 to 10 minutes for questions, and plan your presentation with the time limit in mind. Practice your presentation several times so that you are sure you can get it done within the time constraints. It is common to have only 20 to 30 minutes for your presentation; thus, you will have to focus on the most important points that lead to maximum application of your findings.

What Are Your Objectives?

Design your presentation so that your research results are presented logically. Most research presentations are brief, and thus, you will have to focus on those points that are the most important to get across. A suggested outline for a podium presentation is as follows:
- An introduction to the problem or clinical issue
- The purpose or primary aim of the research and the associated research question
- Design of the study, including a description of the intervention, the measured outcomes, the sampling strategy, and information about the measurement instruments
- The findings from the study, including the type of statistical analysis and the major results
- A discussion of the results, including the major limitations, as well as the most important findings for clinical practice
- Implications for future research and for clinical practice

Develop an outline of the presentation and then add the major points under each element of the outline and, finally, the specific content that you want to present for each major point. Do not write a "speech," but rather create a detailed outline for your reference during the presentation. This detailed outline can serve as a basis for any visuals that you develop to support your presentation.

Often, the introduction is the most difficult part to develop, and waiting until a good introduction occurs to you may delay development of your presentation. Creating an outline for the overall presentation first may help you create an introduction; thus, forge ahead with development of the body of the presentation and develop the introduction later. Statistics about the breadth of the

Overcoming Presentation Fear

Presentation anxiety is considered the most common phobia; if you are anxious about your podium presentation, you are not alone. Some simple things can be done, however, to reduce your fear and present your research in a professional way.

- Preparation and practice are keys to a calm presentation. The more comfortable you are with your content, the more comfortable you will be in front of an audience.
- Get to the room early, and check out the environment and equipment. Anxiety is enhanced by feeling out of control; when you are familiar with the presentation environment and you feel in control, your anxiety will be reduced. Make sure that your audiovisual support is working, that your notes are organized, and that you know the layout of the room. Immediately before the presentation, step outside and "walk off" some of the nervous energy that you feel.
- Use eye contact to your advantage. Pick a friendly face in the first few rows, and focus on them until you are feeling relaxed in front of the group.
- Do not apologize for your lack of experience, discomfort, or any other aspect of the presentation. Apologizing is a sign of a novice presenter, and the audience will have less confidence in your presentation.
- Your most anxious time is likely right before the presentation begins. As you are introduced, breathe deeply, and focus on relaxing your shoulders and neck. When it is your turn to talk, use assertive body language, and stride to the podium with your head up. If you look confident, you will feel confident.
- Do not feel that you have to speak the moment you reach the podium. Take a moment to breathe, scan the audience, and smile. When you are composed, begin speaking.
- If your voice shakes, do not focus on it, and let it work out as you talk. It is highly unlikely that the audience will notice the quiver in your voice.
- Your goal should be to control your anxiety, not completely remove all tension. A small amount of apprehension keeps you on your toes and actually adds energy to your presentation. Keep in mind that even seasoned speakers get nervous; they have learned to control it, and you can, too.

problem are good attention grabbers, as are personal stories about your experience with the issue or quotes from others. Avoid using unrelated jokes or clichés to introduce your presentation, but focus on interesting anecdotes that are directly related to your topic.

Plan to link the major elements of the presentation together with logical transition statements. The relationship between each stage of your research should be clear to the listener. The conclusion should summarize the overall importance of your study, the main concepts that you have discussed and the major implications for practice. Plan the conclusion with a goal of maximum retention of the most important parts of your research.

YOUR PROFESSIONAL CONTRIBUTION: PLANNING FOR PUBLICATION

Poster and podium presentations reach an audience that goes beyond your organization. Still, the number who can learn and use your findings is limited to those who are physically present. Publication in a professional journal reaches the largest target audience and is a reachable goal even for novice researchers.

Your first step should be to find an appropriate journal. Decide on this before the article is written so that you can tailor the manuscript to the journal's specific readership. Review several articles from the journals that you are considering before finalizing your choice. Then check the masthead of the journal or the journal's Web site for author directions. These are generally straightforward and are labeled "directions for authors" or "authors' guidelines." Follow them carefully in preparing and submitting your manuscript. Table 11-2 describes the most common elements of a research manuscript if specifics are not provided by the journal.

Find a journal that has a clearly defined focus that matches the focus of your research. If you are unsure whether your research fits, send an abstract to the editor, asking for feedback about the appropriateness of your work for publication. Do not expect an acceptance at this stage—the editor will almost certainly want to see the entire article—but you can avoid unnecessary rejections if you are sure upfront that the topic is of interest.

If the editor responds negatively, do not be discouraged. The journal may have recently published a similar work or may have multiple submissions on your topic. If one journal turns you down, move on to the next journal that you have considered. Be persistent, using the feedback from each editor to improve your manuscript. Resist the urge to submit to more than one journal at the same time, however. It is possible you could have more than one journal accept your work, and retracting an article after acceptance is undesirable.

Table 11-2   Anatomy of a Research Manuscript

Element	Contents	Considerations
Abstract	Summary of purpose and research question Overview of methods and procedures Major results Implications of the results General conclusions drawn	It is generally written *after* the manuscript is complete. It should be 300 words or less. It reports the most important parts of the study and can stand alone as a description.
Introduction	Detailed statement of the problem Relevance to clinical practice Brief review of the most relevant literature Theoretical framework for the study Specific purpose of the study, research question, and hypotheses (if appropriate)	It provides the context for the research question. The problem and purpose should be in the first few paragraphs. Limit the literature review to the most relevant sources.
Methods and Procedures	Specific study design and rationale for selection Sampling strategy, including selection criteria and method Description of sample, including sample size Measurement methods with documentation of reliability, validity, and procedures	If a well-known measurement and/or treatment are used, then the description can be less detailed. Diagrams and photographs can clarify procedures for intervention or measurement. Provide a description and references only for unique statistical tests.

Table 11-2 Anatomy of a Research Manuscript *(continued)*

Element	Contents	Considerations
Methods and Procedures *(continued)*	Procedures for implementation of the treatment and placebo Data collection and analysis procedures	
Results	Textual description of the statistical tests Tables and figures that summarize the results Decisions for each hypothesis	Tables and figures should not duplicate the text. The information presented in each should be unique. This is a section for reporting only; discussion of the findings comes later.
Discussion	Interpretation of statistical results Discussion of clinical relevance of the findings Contribution of the results to practice Comparison of results with previous works of others Discuss study limitations and strengths Suggest areas for further study	You can express opinions here. Commentary should not reiterate results but expand on them and relate findings to practical uses.
References	A list of all references cited in the manuscript	

For more depth and detail, try these resources:

Albarran, J., and J. Scholes. 2005. How to get published: Seven easy steps. *Nursing in Critical Care* 10: 72–8.

Baggott, I., and J. Bagott. 2001. Talk the talk: Overcome your fear of public speaking. *Nursing Spectrum.* 2:12–13.

Carroll-Johnson, R. 2001. Submitting a manuscript for review. *Clinical Journal of Oncology Nursing* 5(3 Suppl): 13–16.

Korner, A. 2004. *Guide to Publishing a Scientific Paper.* Hamden, CT: Bioscript Press.

DeBehnke, D., J. Kline, and R. Shih. 2001. Research fundamentals: Choosing an appropriate journal, manuscript preparation, and interaction with editors. *Academic Emergency Medicine* 8: 844–50.

Evans, M. 2000. Polished, professional presentation: Unlocking design elements. *Journal of Continuing Education in Nursing* 31: 213–8.

Heyman, B., and P. Conin. 2005. Writing for publication: Adapting academic work into articles. *British Journal of Nursing* 14: 400–4.

Hundley, V. 2002. Research notes: How do you decide where to send an article for publication? *Nursing Standard* 16: 21.

Portney, L., and R. Craik. 1998. Sharing your research: Platform and poster presentations. *PT Magazine* 6: 72–81.

Siwek, J., J. Gourlay, D. Slawson, and A. Shaughnessy. 2002. How to write an evidence-based clinical review article. *American Family Physician* 65: 251–8.

Smith, M. 2000. Public speaking survival strategies. *Journal of Emergency Nursing* 26: 166–8.

Sullivan, E. 2002. Top 10 reasons a manuscript is rejected. *Journal of Professional Nursing* 18: 1–2.

www.kumc.edu/SAH/OTEd/jradel/Poster_Presentations/PstrStart.html

www.presentersonline.com/tutorials/powerpoint/slides/shtml

The review process takes from 4 to 12 weeks. Expect that you may be asked for revisions—some of them substantial—before full acceptance. Even the most seasoned authors make revisions to assure that the article meets the expectations of peer reviewers and editors; thus, do not take editorial comments personally. Use each piece of feedback as guidance for improving your writing and your work.

A note is in order about converting academic papers to a publishable manuscript. Considerable condensing is required while maintaining the key substance and meaning of your work. Specifically, the literature review will be substantially shorter for an article, with a focus on the most relevant citations. To keep the literature review reasonable, do not include any statements that reflect common knowledge in the field or that contribute nothing unique to the study. The writing style should be focused on clarity of expression, using active voice and simplicity of language. Organize the information logically, and take care to remain objective.

SUMMARY

Clinical research in practice requires tremendous effort on the part of the bedside scientist. Although it is a laudable goal to change practice based on empirical evidence generated within the organization, the contribution of knowledge to the field is only complete when your research has been communicated to a larger audience. This may be through posters or presentations at conferences or through publication in a peer reviewed journal. It is only through communication to a broader audience that true changes in practice—generated by clinicians and based on evidence—can occur.

Glossary

Abstract: A summary of a research study that includes a description of the most important aspects of the study (e.g., purpose, subjects, methods, results, and discussion); usually between 100 and 500 words and used for poster, podium, and manuscript submissions.

Alpha: Level of statistical significance, preset by the researcher.

Analysis of variance (ANOVA): A statistical test used to compare means of three or more groups.

Attrition: Loss of subjects after the study has begun.

Audit trail: Documentation of steps and decisions made about design and analysis in a qualitative study; enables the reader to judge internal validity.

Bias: Alternative explanations for the findings of a study; any element that is not part of the study but influences the outcome.

Blinding: A blind *review* is an unbiased review of a manuscript by a professional peer who is unaware of authorship. A blinded *study* is one in which the researcher, data collectors, and/or subjects are unaware of whether they are in the experimental or control group.

Bracketing: In qualitative studies, the process of explicitly identifying the researcher's biases so that they can be set aside during the study; a measure to control internal validity.

Case/control study: A research design often used in retrospective studies that involves comparing some characteristic of cases (those with a condition) to matched controls (those without the condition but who are similar in key ways).

Categorical variable: A variable that can be measured by categorizing the subject's characteristics into mutually exclusive classifications (e.g., ethnicity).

Central tendency: Descriptive statistics that represent a "typical" case, commonly represented by the mean, the median, and the mode.

Chi-square test: A test used to determine whether two categorical variables have an association.

Coding: The process of analyzing qualitative data by identifying patterns or themes.

Coefficient alpha: A statistic that represents internal reliability of a measurement instrument.

Coefficient of correlation: A number that represents the direction and strength of a correlation.

Cohort study: A study of a specific group of subjects over time.

Confidentiality: Measures put into place to assure that subject data, including identity, are protected from unauthorized access.

Consent form: A written agreement that lays out the expectations and conditions of a study for review by potential subjects before the start of an experiment; subjects must sign a consent form before they can be in an experiment.

Constant comparison: A method of qualitative analysis in which new data are compared with data that have already been collected to determine and refine the coding scheme.

Content validity: The extent to which the content of an instrument reflects what it is intended to measure.

Continuous variable: A variable that can take on a value anywhere on a scale.

Control group: The group in a randomized control trial that receives no treatment or a standard treatment; outcomes in the control group are compared with those in the experimental group to see if the treatment had an effect.

Convenience sample: A sample selected because of its accessibility and availability to the researcher; a sample chosen other than randomly.

Criterion-related validity: The extent to which performance on a measurement instrument correlates with performance on some predetermined, external criterion.

Cross-sectional study: A study based on measuring some characteristic in several groups at a specific point in time.

Dependent variable: A variable that the experimenter analyzes to determine whether there is an effect of the independent variable; in cause-and-effect, the dependent variable is the effect.

Descriptive statistics: Statistics that summarize research data.

Double-blind study: An experiment in which neither the researcher nor the subject knows who is getting the treatment.

Effect size: The magnitude of the difference between the experimental and control group, irrespective of statistical significance; effect size determines whether results are clinically meaningful.

Electronic database: Bibliographic data files that can be searched for a literature review.

Emergent design: A characteristic of qualitative study in which design decisions are made as the study unfolds.

Ethnography: A type of qualitative study that involves extended observation and analysis of the culture of a group; derived from the anthropology field.

Evidence-based practice: Careful and systematic review and use of current best evidence in decision making that takes into consideration clinician expertise and patient considerations and preferences.

Exclusion criteria: Objective characteristics that would make a subject unsuitable for a study.

Ex post facto design: Research conducted after a phenomenon of interest has already occurred.

Experimental design: A scientific method in which a treatment is applied to a randomly selected group and an outcome of interest is compared with a group that does not receive the treatment.

Experimental group: The subjects who receive the treatment in an experimental design.

External validity: The degree to which findings from a study sample can be applied to a larger or different population.

Extraneous variable: A variable that is not part of the formal study design but nevertheless has an impact on the outcome; internal validity requires that extraneous variables are controlled.

Face validity: The extent to which a measurement instrument "looks like" it represents the underlying concepts.

Focus group interview: A group interview of individuals designed to answer specific questions.

Frequency distribution: A table of the frequency of each score in a set of scores.

Frequency histogram: A graph that displays the frequency of scores as bars.

Frequency polygon: A graph that displays the frequency of scores by connecting points representing them above each score.

Generalizability: The degree to which population characteristics can be inferred from a sample.

Hawthorne effect: A change in subject behavior as a result of their awareness of the study.

Hypothesis: A statistically testable statement of a relationship between two variables.

Inclusion criteria: Preset, objective criteria that describe in detail the characteristics of subjects that are appropriate for an experiment.

Independent variable: A variable of interest that the researcher manipulates in an experiment; the treatment or intervention; in cause and effect, the independent variable is the cause.

Inferential statistics: Statistics used to determine whether the results from studying a sample can be inferred to a population; typically used to separate effects of the independent variable from those caused by chance (sampling error) alone.

Institutional review board (IRB): A formalized group that reviews research proposals to determine whether they meet ethical standards for protection of human subjects.

Internal validity: The extent to which alternative explanations for the results of an experiment have been accounted for, eliminated, or controlled.

Interrater reliability: A measure of the level of agreement between two raters who are measuring or categorizing the same variables.

Level of measurement: A classification of measures reflecting the nature of a measurement that dictates the kind of analysis that can be used; the four levels are nominal, ordinal, interval, and ratio.

Likert scale: A measure in which subjects are asked to rate their level of agreement or disagreement with a statement using a number.

Line graph: A graph used to plot data showing the relationship between independent and dependent variables in an experiment.

Longitudinal study: A study conducted over time.

Mean: The arithmetic average of a set of scores.

Measurement: The quantification of some characteristic of a subject.

Median: The middle score in a set of scores that has been ordered from lowest to highest.

Meta-analysis: A study of the composite effect size of multiple studies; integrates the findings of several studies on the same subject.

Mixed-method research: A study that uses elements of both quantitative and qualitative research.

Mode: The score that occurs most frequently in a set of scores.

N/n: Size of the sample or population that was studied; a capital N generally indicates a population, and a lower case n indicates a sample.

Negative skew: A graph that has scores bunching up toward the positive end of the graph.

Normal curve: A graph with a bell-shaped curve in which most of the scores are clustered around the mean. The scores become less frequent the farther they are from the mean.

Null hypothesis: The prediction that the independent variable will have no effect on the dependent variable in an experiment.

Operational definition: An objective definition of a variable in terms of its quantitative measurement.

P value: A calculated value that represents the probability that results are due to sampling error. In general, p values of less than 0.05 are considered statistically significant.

Peer review: Review of a completed research study by a professional expert in the field.

Percentile: The score at or below which a particular percentage of scores fall.

Phenomenology: A type of qualitative study in which the researcher studies the responses of subjects who have all experienced the same phenomenon.

Pie graph: A descriptive graph that represents data as percentages of a pie.

Population: All individuals who are of interest in a given experiment.

Positive skew: A graph that has scores bunching up toward the negative end of the scale.

Post hoc test: A test run after an omnibus test (such as ANOVA) to identify and quantify specific differences between groups.

Poster session: A session at a professional conference during which many researchers present visual displays of their research; allows for individual interaction with the author.

Power: The ability of a given sample to find a treatment effect if it exists.

Power analysis: Determination of the number of subjects needed to achieve an acceptable level of power.

Psychometric evaluation: Evaluation of the reliability and validity of a measurement instrument.

Purposive sampling: A convenience sample of subjects that is selected based on the researcher's personal judgment about his or her ability to inform the research question.

Qualitative research: Collection and analysis of data collected through naturalistic methods via observation or by soliciting subjects' words.

Quantitative research: Collection and analysis of data that are measured or categorized as numerical values.

Quasiexperimental design: An experiment in which a treatment is applied and an outcome of interest is measured, but in which subjects are selected or assigned to groups other than randomly.

Random assignment: A mathematical process of assigning subjects to the experimental or treatment group using random methods.

Random sampling: Sample selection procedure in which every member of the population has an equal and independent probability of selection.

Range: A statistic representing the difference between the highest and lowest scores in a data set.

Reliability: The capacity of an instrument to measure consistently the true score of an individual; when variations occur in responses, they are due to differences in the subjects, not to variability within the instrument.

Replication: The intentional repetition of an experiment to determine whether similar results are found.

Research question: The objective of a study; a statement of the information the researcher hopes to find.

Sample: A subset of a population of interest that is selected or recruited to participate in a study.

Sampling error: Variation in the data that is attributable to the way the sample is drawn from the population; also called standard error.

Saturation: A standard for sample size in a qualitative study in which the researcher judges that no new information is being generated.

Scatter plot: A graph of a correlation relationship.

Standard deviation: A statistic representing the degree of distribution of a set of scores around the mean; the average distance of the data points from the mean.

Statistical significance: A low probability (usually less than 5%) that the results of a research study are due to chance factors rather than to the independent variable.

Statistics: Mathematical techniques used to summarize research data or to determine whether the data support the researcher's hypothesis.

Subject: A single participant in an experiment.

Survey research: Research in which data are gathered directly from subjects about attitudes, perceptions, beliefs, or attributes.

Test statistic: A numerical value that represents the differences between groups when sampling error is taken into account.

Test–retest reliability: Stability of an instrument over time, measured by correlating the responses of a group of subjects on an instrument at two different time periods.

Thick description: Detailed description of the context and environment of a qualitative study.

Time series design: An experimental design in which a baseline is measured in a group of subjects, an intervention applied, and then sequential measures are taken over time.

Triangulation: The use of three or more sources to confirm conclusions in a qualitative analysis.

Validity: The degree to which a measurement instrument represents what it purports to measure.

A Sample Informed Consent Form

STUDY TITLE: The Effects of Parent–Physician Relationships on the Recovery of Hospitalized Children with Bronchiolitis
(Parent Consent)

PRINCIPAL INVESTIGATOR:

Scott M. Brenner, MD
Medical Director, Inpatient Pediatrics
Lehigh Valley Hospital
Cedar Crest Boulevard and I-78
Allentown, Pennsylvania, 18105
██████████████

PURPOSE:

You are being asked to take part in a research study because your child has been hospitalized with Bronchiolitis. The purpose of this research study is to understand how both 1) the anxiety of parents, and 2) their relationship with the doctors and nurses may affect the course of their child's illness.

STUDY PROCEDURES:

If you agree to be part of the study, the following things will happen:

1. A validated bronchiolitis scoring sheet to evaluate the severity of your child's condition will be completed daily by the physician caring for your child.

2. You will complete a 40-item questionnaire that asks about your anxiety level and a six-item questionnaire asking about your child's hospitalization and your previous experience with hospitals at the time of your entrance into the study. This should take about 15 to 20 minutes of your time.

3. Each day after that, you will complete the first 20 items of the first questionnaire again to evaluate your level of anxiety on that day and two extra questions regarding your child's care. This should take about 10 minutes of your time.

4. Once completed, your questionnaires will be placed in a sealed envelope and will not be seen by the study team or anyone providing care to your child. The information will later be entered into a computer database and you will only be identified by a study identification number and not your name.

You do not have to participate in this study. Also, you can stop being in the study at any time. Stopping or not being in the study will not upset anyone. The doctors and staff will keep taking care of your child and interacting with you as they normally would.

The doctors and staff will answer your questions about this study at any time.

BENEFITS:

You may or may not receive any direct benefit from participating in this study. By better understanding your attitudes and anxiety about your child's hospitalization, as well as how you interact with your child's doctors and nurses, the researchers are hoping to provide better care to pediatric patients.

ALTERNATIVES TO STUDY PARTICIPATION:

There is no obligation to participate in the study and you may choose not to.

RISKS AND DISCOMFORTS:

There is minimal risk to you as a participant in this research study. It may be stressful to reflect on your feelings during your child's hospitalization.

COMPENSATION FOR INJURY OR ILLNESS:

In the unlikely event of any injury or illness resulting from your participation in this study, treatment can be provided by Lehigh Valley Hospital, the costs of which will be charged to you or your insurance company. Lehigh Valley Hospital will not be responsible for providing either financial compensation or free medical treatment as a result of your participation in this study. By signing this informed consent document and allowing your child to be in this study, you do not lose any of your legal rights that you or your child would otherwise have.

AUTHORIZATION FOR RELEASE OF HEALTH INFORMATION AND CONFIDENTIALITY STATEMENT:

In order to participate in this research study, you must authorize the release of your child's health information related to and used for purposes of this research study. The principal investigator is responsible for overseeing the use and disclosure of your child's health information data, and your responses to the questionnaires. Any information about your child and his or her treatment obtained from this research—including your child's medical history, laboratory data, and findings on physical examination, biopsy and surgery—will be kept confidential and never identified in any report. Should results of this study be reported in medical journals or at meetings, the names of all participants will remain anonymous. Only authorized representatives, including the study personnel, the federal Food and Drug Administration (FDA), the Department of Health and Human Services (DHHS), and this hospital's institutional review board (IRB), will have access to your child's medical records relating to this research; all information examined will be coded and kept confidential. However, because of this potential need to release information to outside parties, absolute confidentiality cannot be guaranteed.

Your child's study-related health information may be re-disclosed by any of the organizations listed above and may no longer be protected. This re-disclosure would be done only in your child's best interests; the agencies listed above monitor clinical research to ensure studies are conducted appropriately and ethically.

This authorization to release your child's health information is effective from (the date you sign this consent form) until the submitted study results are statistically analyzed. After receiving authorization, your child's current and past medical records will be reviewed to ensure he or she is eligible to participate in this study, and your child's health status is accurately reflected in the information reported for the study.

You and your child will be allowed to participate only after you give your authorization to release your child's health information. You may withdraw your authorization at any time, in writing, by notifying Dr. Scott Brenner, Lehigh Valley Hospital, Cedar Crest Boulevard and I-78, Allentown, PA, 18105. Your withdrawal of authorization will be effective upon receipt of this written notice and will allow the investigator to use only the health information that was gathered up until your withdrawal to the extent necessary to preserve the integrity of (follow through and properly complete) the research study. Your withdrawal from participation in the study itself, as discussed below, will automatically withdraw your authorization to use your child's health information data and your responses to the questionnaires.

ACCESS TO YOUR MEDICAL/RESEARCH RECORDS:

The Health Insurance Portability and Accountability Act's (HIPAA's) Standards for Privacy of Individually Identifiable Health Information grants patients and their parents the right to review their medical records. If your child is a participant in a research study, you understand that you may be denied access to his or her medical records for the period of time he or she participates in this research study. If you are denied access, after completion of the research study, you may again have access to your child's medical records.

OPTION OF WITHDRAWAL WITHOUT PREJUDICE:

Your decision whether or not to participate in this study is voluntary and will not affect your child's medical care. Also, you understand that if for any reason, you wish to withdraw from this study, you are free to do so at any time. If you decide to participate in the study, the researchers are required by federal regulations (45 CFR 46) to have you read the following statement and sign your name below it.

I have been given the chance to ask questions and had them answered to my satisfaction. I consent to take part in this study. I understand that if I have further questions about the study, I may contact Scott Brenner, MD, at ▇▇▇▇▇▇▇▇. I understand that if I want information regarding my or my child's rights as a research participant, I may contact Thomas Wasser, PhD, institutional review board (IRB) administrator at Lehigh Valley Hospital by telephoning ▇▇▇▇▇▇▇▇. I will receive a signed copy of this consent form to keep for my records.

Parent/Guardian Signature   Date

Printed Name of Parent/Guardian

Physician/Investigator Signature (or Designee/Person Obtaining Consent) Date

---

Printed Name of Physician/Investigator (or Designee/Person Obtaining Consent)

Witness Signature   Date

Printed Name of Witness

Disclaimer: This consent form should be used only as an example of what one organization has done to meet their institutional review board (IRB), HIPAA, and legal requirements. It is not meant to serve as a standard. Each organization will need to meet their own IRB, HIPAA and legal requirements. Used by permission.

A Survey for a Bedside Science Project

PATIENT EVALUATION OF HOSPITALIZATION FOR RADICAL PROSTATECTOMY

Patient Name _____ *Prostatectomy Date:* _____ *Today's Date:* _____

Read the following:: *"Recently, you had a radical prostatectomy. This survey will tell us how you felt about your pre hospital education and hospital care by your doctors and nursing staff. By answering these questions, you may benefit other patients who will have radical prostatectomies in the future.* **Whether or not you choose to answer these questions is up to you.** *This survey will take approximately 5 - 7 minutes to complete."*

HOW SATISFIED WERE YOU WITH:	Very Dissatisfied	Somewhat Dissatisfied	Neutral	Somewhat Satisfied	Very Satisfied
1. Your hospital stay?	1 ☐	2 ☐	3 ☐	4 ☐	5 ☐
2. The information you received about your hospital stay **prior to being admitted** to the hospital.	1 ☐	2 ☐	3 ☐	4 ☐	5 ☐
3. The information your **PHYSICIAN** provided regarding your hospitalization and illness throughout your hospital stay?	1 ☐	2 ☐	3 ☐	4 ☐	5 ☐
4. The information your **NURSE** provided regarding your hospitalization and illness throughout your hospital stay?	1 ☐	2 ☐	3 ☐	4 ☐	5 ☐

5. The education and training you received **by nursing staff** for the following:	Very Dissatisfied	Somewhat Dissatisfied	Satisfied	Somewhat Satisfied	Very Satisfied
A) Changing your leg bag	1 ☐	2 ☐	3 ☐	4 ☐	5 ☐
B) Proper foley catheter care and hygiene	1 ☐	2 ☐	3 ☐	4 ☐	5 ☐
C) Caring for your drain (answer only if you had one)	1 ☐	2 ☐	3 ☐	4 ☐	5 ☐

6. Select the response that best describes **how well** the pain medication you received following surgery controlled your pain:

THE PAIN MEDICATION RELIEVED MY PAIN:

Always	Usually	Sometimes	Rarely	Never
1 ☐	2 ☐	3 ☐	4 ☐	5 ☐

7. Based on the **PAIN SCALE** (on a scale of 0 – 10, with 0 being NO PAIN and 10 being WORST POSSIBLE PAIN)

A) Describe your **incisional pain** when it was at its worst while in the hospital. (This would be separate from any discomforts related to catheters, tubes and/or hospital beds).

No Pain   Moderate Pain   Worst Possible Pain

0 ☐ 1 ☐ 2 ☐ 3 ☐ 4 ☐ 5 ☐ 6 ☐ 7 ☐ 8 ☐ 9 ☐ 10 ☐

B) Describe your **incisional pain after** you were medicated:

0 ☐ 1 ☐ 2 ☐ 3 ☐ 4 ☐ 5 ☐ 6 ☐ 7 ☐ 8 ☐ 9 ☐ 10 ☐

	Not Prepared	Somewhat Unprepared	Neutral	Somewhat Prepared	Completely Prepared
8. How ready or prepared did you feel to go home?	1 ☐	2 ☐	3 ☐	4 ☐	5 ☐
9. On your day of discharge, how prepared did you feel to **CARE for yourself** at home?	1 ☐	2 ☐	3 ☐	4 ☐	5 ☐

10. Were you discharged to home with **HOME CARE** services?   YES ☐   NO ☐

11. Tell me the top three things we could have done to **improve** your stay:
    1)
    2)
    3)

12. Tell me the top three things that you **appreciated** during your stay:
    1)
    2)
    3)

Revised 10/28/02

Appraisal of the Evidence: Reviewing a Published Article

Chang, B.H., A. Hendricks, U. Zhao, J.A. Rothendler, J.S. LoCastro, and M.T. Slawsky. 2005. A relaxation response randomized trial on patients with chronic heart failure. *Journal of Cardiopulmonary Rehabilitation* 25: 149–157. Reprinted with permission of Lippincott, Williams and Wilkins.

In 1997, relaxation techniques (usually meditation) were the most commonly reported complementary and alternative therapy.[1] In the relaxation response (RR) state, individuals evoke a quiet body and calm mind with physiologic effects opposite to the fight-or-flight stress response.[2–4] Unlike the stress response, the RR does not occur spontaneously. It can be elicited by various simple, noninvasive techniques.[3]

Physiologic and psychological benefits of the RR have been reported in the literature. Physiologic effects triggered by the RR include decreased metabolism, oxygen consumption, carbon dioxide elimination, respiratory rate, heart rate, minute ventilation, and arterial blood lactate.[2–4] All these responses appear to involve a reduction in the activity of the sympathetic nervous system and have a favorable impact on myocardial oxygen supply and demand. Psychologic effects of the RR include lower levels of anxiety, hostility, and depression.[5–8] Benefits of the RR have been reported for various medical conditions, including hypertension and coronary artery disease.[9–11]

Literature Review Critique

The literature review for this article begins in the introduction. The authors provide support for the importance of the study by documenting the severity of the problem and by presenting evidence that makes a logical link between the intervention and potential outcomes. The literature serves to provide a basis for believing that the intervention can, indeed, have an effect on this problem. The evidence basis for the intervention is slim—only two small studies were found—and thus, there is a gap in knowledge relative to this intervention, making it a good subject for a randomized trial.

The effect of the RR on chronic heart failure (CHF), a highly prevalent, costly condition associated with hypertension, coronary artery disease, anxiety, and depression, has not been well studied. A major target in CHF treatment is relief of adverse responses resulting from overextension of the sympathetic nervous system. The RR intervention, with its reduction in the activity of the sympathetic nervous system, has the potential to improve symptoms and quality of life (QOL) of CHF patients. With the disease progress of CHF characterized as a fairly long period of illness punctuated by crises, any one of which might prove fatal, it is particularly important to identify interventions that can benefit the spiritual and emotional QOL of CHF patients.

Two very small pilot studies reported that meditation and imagery training improved psychologic well-being, QOL, and walking distance in certain time, but not exercise performance or dyspnea.[12,13] Here, we report a randomized clinical trial, which included a qualitative substudy, to evaluate the effect of an RR intervention on CHF patients. The results of the qualitative substudy are published elsewhere.[14] This article reports the quantitative results.

METHOD

Study Design

This randomized clinical trial included three study groups: RR, cardiac education (EDU), and usual care (UC). The EDU group served as an alternative intervention and was also used to control for possible effects associated with group meetings and patients' expectations for improvement. The institutional review boards at the Veterans Affairs (VA) Boston Healthcare System (BHS) and the Edith Nourse Rogers Memorial Veterans Hospital at Bedford approved this study.

Design Critique

The authors apply an experimental design, essentially comparing the intervention group to two control groups. One of the control groups receives usual care, and the second control group gets an alternative treatment—a cardiac education program. The latter group helps control the Hawthorne effect, or changes in behavior due to the simple act of being in a study. This is a particularly strong characteristic of this study, as it controls for potential treatment effects, the basis for one of the most common criticisms of simple randomized controlled trials.

Inclusion and Exclusion Criteria

The study targeted ambulatory CHF patients (ICD-9 codes 428, 428.0, 428.1, and 428.9 listed in VA databases) who visited the VA BHS during the study period and had (1) moderate symptom severity (New York Heart Association [NYHA] classification II or III) and (2) left ventricular ejection fraction (LVEF) less than or equal to 40%. Exclusion criteria were (1) participation in a rehabilitation program with exercise training or an education group within the prior year, (2) currently practicing RR or any form of meditation, or (3) cognitively impaired (Mini-Mental State Examination > 24 points).

Criteria and Question Critique

Both inclusion and exclusion criteria were applied to this experiment, and the criteria are very detailed and objective. This is a strong point. What is missing so far, however? By this point in the article, it is usual to have specifically presented the purpose of the study and an explicit research question. Although both the purpose and the question can be inferred from the information already presented, it would be a stronger research report if these two key elements appeared in the first few paragraphs.

Patient Recruitment and Study Participants Characteristics

Patients were recruited between April 2000 and June 2002 from the CHF, cardiac, and primary care clinics at the VA BHS. A total of 482 CHF patients with LVEF less than or equal to 40% were screened in clinic (see Figure A3-1). Among them, 315 (65%) declined, and 124 (26%) consented to participate. The main reason for declining was "lived too far away." A small percentage (N = 36, 7%) of patients screened were found ineligible. Seven patients did not complete screening and could not be reached afterward. Of the 124 patients who consented, 31% (N = 39) did not come back for baseline assessments; the remaining 85 patients underwent baseline assessments and were considered enrolled. Patient recruitment by telephone from February to April 2001 yielded another 10 enrollees. Recruitment details are described elsewhere.[15] Total enrollment was 95 (Figure A3-1).

Despite a high refusal rate, there was no strong evidence of selection bias. The characteristics of enrolled patients and those who refused were similar (i.e., no statistical difference): gender (both 99% men), race (85% vs. 84% white), LVEF (31.2% vs. 31.7%), and CHF medications (angiotensin-converting enzyme inhibitors: 82% vs. 75%, [beta]-blockers: 78% vs. 71%). Enrolled patients

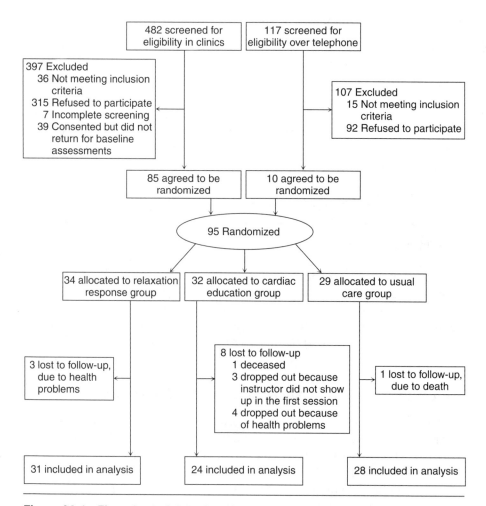

Figure A3-1 Flow chart of the relaxation response randomized trial.

were slightly younger (70 vs. 73 years old) and lived closer to the study site (23 vs. 30 miles).

Randomization

After enrollment and completion of baseline outcome assessments (see the Study Measures section), patients were randomly assigned to one of the study groups according to random numbers generated by a computer program. The RR, EDU, and UC groups numbered 34, 32, and 29, respectively.

Sampling Critique

The authors describe the recruitment process in great detail, providing the numbers that help us evaluate whether sampling bias or attrition may have affected this study. The researchers admit to the high refusal rate but also take pains to exclude selection bias by statistically comparing the key characteristics of subjects who agreed to be in the study to those who refused. No difference was found, and thus, it can be concluded that the refusal rate did not affect the ultimate sample in a systematic way. Subjects were assigned to groups randomly, and thus, a strong case can be made that any variables that might affect the outcome are evenly distributed among all groups. It would have been helpful to know if a power analysis was conducted prospectively so that the reader could decide if the sample had sufficient power to detect group differences.

Study Intervention

Patients randomized to RR were requested to attend 15 weekly 90-minute group sessions to learn 8 techniques to elicit the RR (breathing awareness; mental repetition of a word, sound, phrase, or prayer; mindfulness meditation; guided body scan; progressive muscle relaxation; guided countdown; autogenic; and guided imagery). A tape with the mental repetition, body scan, and mindfulness meditation was purchased from The Mind Body Medical Institute.[16] Instructions for the other techniques were recorded on another 3 tapes by the study clinical psychologist using a modified script from a stress reduction book, whose author gave written permission to record the scripts.[17] Patients were also taught short versions of relaxation exercises (minis) involving focused breathing techniques. Trained clinical psychologists, with the aid of these tapes, instructed patient groups on each technique. Patients were asked to practice at home twice a day by using the tapes (each technique lasts about 20 minutes) provided and to keep a diary of the frequency of practice. Home practice of once or twice a day was recommended by The Mind Body Medical Institute. We chose twice per day to increase the likelihood of the intervention effect.

Cardiac Education

The EDU patients were requested to attend 15 weekly 90-minute cardiac education lectures. This ongoing education program was organized by the Cardiac Rehabilitation Education Program at the VA BHS. Speakers were experts on medical, pharmaceutical, lifestyle, nutrition, and psychosocial issues affecting people with heart disease. The RR training was not included in the EDU.

Procedure Critique

The procedures for each intervention group—both the intervention of interest and the cardiac education—are described in detail. This controls the possibility that differences in the way the intervention was applied could have been responsible for any differences that may have been discovered between groups. This section supports replication of the study to see whether these results can be achieved with other samples in other settings.

Usual Care

The UC patients were not requested to attend any group sessions. They were expected to complete the study outcome assessments at baseline and the follow-up assessment.

Study Measures

Outcomes included objective measures of exercise capacity and subjective measures of QOL. The Minnesota Living with Heart Failure (MLwHF) Questionnaire, with physical and emotional subscales, was used to measure disease-specific QOL; lower scores indicated better health. The Functional Assessment of Chronic Illness Therapy—Spiritual Well-Being, with peace and faith subscales, measured the spiritual domain of QOL; higher scores indicate better spiritual QOL. Both QOL measures have good validity and reliability[18,19] and are commonly used to evaluate treatment and intervention effects.[20,21] Study participants self-administered these QOL questionnaires at baseline when they were recruited in the clinic. The follow-up questionnaires were handed out to the RR and EDU group participants at their last session of the 15-week intervention program or no later than 19 weeks after the baseline assessment for patients who missed some of the weekly group sessions. The follow-up questionnaires were mailed out to the UC group participants. Participants returned the complete questionnaires when they came to the follow-up bicycle exercise test (see below) or by mail. Because of the nature of the study intervention, participants were not blinded to their group assignments.

Peak oxygen consumption (VO_2max) is commonly used to evaluate exercise capacity with higher values indicating greater capacity.[22,23] Peak VO_2 L/min/kg was measured using a cardiopulmonary bicycle exercise test performed in the exercise laboratory in the VA BHS. An incremental exercise test was performed until volitional fatigue or symptoms of myocardial ischemia ap-

Measurement Critique

The measures used in this study are described thoroughly, as are measurement procedures. This is a strong point, as it means that differences between groups are not likely due to differences in the way the measurements were collected. It is particularly helpful that the authors tell us which end of each scale is better and which is worse; this helps to alleviate confusion later when looking at numerical results. Other strengths include: those who interpreted physiologic measures were blinded as to group assignment, and variables that could represent extraneous variables were collected so that their effects could be quantified. This section overall reflects a very strong measurement plan. One small criticism exists, however—although the authors report that all of the instruments have documented reliability and validity, it would be stronger if the actual reliability and validity statistics were reported. A review of the actual statistics enables the reader to judge the amount of measurement error that may have contributed to the outcome.

peared. Peak oxygen uptake was determined as the highest value recorded during the last 30 seconds of exercise. A cardiologist read test reports to abstract peak VO_2, exercise time, and work load. The exercise physiologist and cardiologist were blinded to patient group assignment.

To adjust for confounding variables, we collected information on comorbidity, social support, special diet, and physical activities. Diagnoses for calculating the Charlson Index[24,25] were obtained from VA administrative files to measure comorbidity. Social support was measured by the Medical Outcomes Study Social Support Survey, a reliable (Cronbach's alpha > 0.90) and valid scale.[26] The Physical Activity Scale for the Elderly, with good reliability and validity,[27] measured the frequency of various physical activities and exercise.

Statistical Analysis

Analyses were based on patient group assignment regardless of compliance with the study protocol (as part of the "intention to treat" principle). Separate regression models were used to estimate the intervention effect on each of the QOL scales and the exercise capacity measures with the change scores between 2 assessments as the dependent variable. Planned pairwise comparisons among the 3 study groups were performed. Because the group comparison was planned prior to the study, type I error adjustment for multiple comparison was not performed.[28] To compare each of the 2 interventions to UC (reference group), the regression model included RR and EDU indicator variables as independent variables. The regression coefficients of these 2 indicator variables are the mean difference in the adjusted change score (adjusting for covariates) between UC and each of RR and EDU groups. The adjusting covariates included variables that were different among the 3 study groups (see "Results" section), and also age and CHF medications that are likely to be associated with the outcome measures. Adjusted mean change scores for each study group were calculated using the mean value of the continuous covariates (e.g., mean age) and the reference group of the dichotomous covariates (e.g., less than college education) applied to the regression coefficients.

RESULTS

Study Attrition

Eighty-three of 95 enrollees completed follow-up questionnaires (31 RR, 24 EDU, and 28 UC), a 13% attrition rate (3 RR, 8 EDU, and 1 UC; see Figure A3-1). Greater EDU attrition reflected 3 patients who claimed the instructor did not show up for the first class. Withdrawals included a death in each of the EDU and UC groups and patients with health problems that prevented group attendance. The 12 patients with missing data on follow-up measures due to dropout were not significantly different from the 83 patients with follow-up measures in demographic characteristics, disease severity, diet, CHF medications, social support, physical activity, and baseline QOL scores ([chi]^2 or t test, p = 0.20).

Baseline Characteristics

Enrolled patients were randomly assigned to a group, but there were significant differences in Spiritual QOL measures at baseline (Table A3-1; N = 95). The UC patients had the lowest baseline scores and EDU had the highest baseline scores in both peace and faith subscale scores. In addition, RR patients were less likely to have a salt-restricted diet and UC patients had the lowest percentage of college graduates. The groups nevertheless had similar baseline scores in the disease-specific QOL measures, MLwHF, age, race, income, disease severity, comorbidity, CHF medications, social support, and physical activity level.

Baseline comparisons among the 3 groups for the 83 patients who had both baseline and follow-up measures (data not shown) reached the same conclusions, further verifying a lack of dropout bias. Our subsequent analysis on change scores between the 2 assessments was based on the 83 patients with both baseline and follow-up assessments.[29]

Analysis I Critique

The planned analysis sounds complicated—and it is—thus, we will wait until we see the actual results to look for helpful numbers. Here, the authors use statistics to show that the subjects who were lost to follow-up were not different than those who stayed in the study. This is an important finding, as it minimizes the effects of attrition. They did, however, discover that the groups were not identical in terms of their baseline measures.

Time Interval Between Assessments

The protocol required follow-up assessments right after the 15-week intervention or no later than 19 weeks after baseline assessment. Most RR and EDU participants did not start the intervention immediately, and some did not attend weekly. Consequently, their follow-up assessments were more than 15 weeks after baseline, giving a longer time interval between the outcome assessments for RR and EDU compared with UC (mean: 169, 155, and 142 days; see Table A3-1).

Some follow-up assessments were also delayed by difficulties in administering the bicycle test (e.g., unavailability of supervising cardiologist, exercise physiologist, or exercise test bicycle). We tried to schedule the follow-up questionnaire assessment to be close to the date of the bicycle test, and thus, delays in the bicycle test affected QOL follow-up assessments. As a result, the time intervals between assessments varied across participants.

QOL Change Score Group Comparison

The mean QOL scores at baseline and the follow-up as well as the change scores for each study group are listed in Table A3-2. Although there was no statistically significant difference among the 3 groups in the crude change scores, there was a trend indicating that RR patients had the best mean change scores, followed by EDU patients and then by UC patients in the emotional subscale of the MLwHF measure (mean of 0.1, 1.1, and 1.7, respectively, with positive values indicating deterioration) and the peace subscale of the spiritual QOL measure (mean of 1.3, -0.5, and -0.4, respectively, with positive values indicating improvement). Given the longer interval between assessments for the intervention groups and difference in the baseline QOL scores, we compared the change scores among the 3 study groups, using a regression model that controlled/adjusted for variables that were different among the 3 groups: baseline QOL scores, education, salt-restricted diet, and time interval between assessments. We also controlled/adjusted for age and CHF medications due to their likely as-

Table A3-1   Patient Characteristics at Baseline

Variable	Study Group, Mean (SD) / n (%)		
	RR (N = 34*)	EDU (N = 32*)	UC (N = 29*)
Demographic characteristics			
Age, y	69.7 (8.9)	68.7 (9.9)	69.2 (10.2)
Race			
White, Non-white (mainly African American)	30, 4 (88%, 12%)	25, 7 (78%. 22%)	23, 6 (79%, 21%)
Education†			
College and above	15 (44%)	19 (59%)	8 (28%)
Disease severity			
LVEF‡	31.1 (6.9)	30.4 (7.7)	32.2 (6.2)
NYHA§: classes II and III	16, 18 (47%, 53%)	18, 12 (60%, 40%)	12, 15 (44%, 56%)
Charlson's Index	3.2 (1.4)	3.3 (1.8)	3.3 (1.5)
Quality of life			
Minnesota Living with Heart Failure (MLwHF)‖			
Physical health	20.5 (10.1)	18.5 (11.2)	22.2 (11.9)
Emotional health	8.2 (7.5)	7.1 (7.2)	8.9 (7.7)
Spiritual scale¶			
Peace†	29.8 (6.9)	31.6 (6.9)	27.1 (7.4)
Faith†,*	13.3 (5.4)	15.0 (3.9)	12.2 (4.9)
Days between assessments#			
Number of days†	169.2 (43.7)	154.5 (43.9)	141.6 (46.2)
>163 days	14 (45%)	11 (46%)	7 (25%)
On salt-restricted diet†			
Yes	21 (62%)	28 (88%)	22 (76%)
Social support	15.0 (6.6)	17.2 (6.3)	17.9 (5.6)
Physical activity	6.0 (3.0)	6.4 (3.3)	5.3 (3.3)
Medication: Taking specified medication			
Ace inhibitors / angiotensin II inhibitors	30 (88%)	30 (94%)	26 (90%)
β-Blockers	26 (76%)	27 (84%)	23 (79%)
Diuretics	22 (65%)	22 (69%)	18 (62%)

*Included all patients with baseline assessments in each study group.
†Statistical significance level for pair comparison among 3 study groups; $P \leq .05$.
‡Left ventricular ejection fraction (LVEF), in percentage.
§New York Heart Association Classification (NYHA), class III has more symptoms than class II, and each of the EDU and UC groups had 2 missing observations.
‖Minnesota Living with Heart Failure measure: MLwHF.
¶Lower scores indicate better health for the disease-specific QOL measure: MLwHF.
#Higher scores indicate better health for the spiritual QOL measure: The Functional Assessment of Chronic Illness Therapy—Spiritual Well-Being Scale.
#Included 83 patients with both assessments: 31 in RR group, 24 in EDU group, and 28 in UC group.

Table A3-2 Baseline, Follow-Up, and Change Scores of Quality-of-Life Measures

	Mean (SD)								
	RR (N = 31)			EDU (N = 24)			UC (N = 28)		
Quality-of-Life Measures*	Baseline	Follow-up	Change Score[†]	Baseline	Follow-up	Change Score[†]	Baseline	Follow-up	Change Score[†]
Disease specific QOL: Minnesota Living with Heart Failure (MLwHF)									
Physical health	19.5 (9.8)	19.3 (12.0)	−0.2 (10.6)	18.0 (10.2)	18.8 (12.3)	0.8 (6.3)	22.6 (12.0)	23.5 (9.4)	0.9 (12.2)
Emotional health	8.1 (7.1)	8.2 (7.8)	0.1 (7.2)	6.9 (7.2)	8.0 (7.3)	1.1 (6.3)	9.3 (7.6)	10.9 (7.2)	1.7 (8.2)
Spiritual scale									
Peace	30.2 (6.3)	31.5 (7.3)	1.3 (4.9)	31.9 (7.0)	31.4 (6.4)	−0.5 (4.5)	26.6 (7.1)	26.2 (4.8)	−0.4 (5.2)
Strength	13.6 (5.4)	14.3 (5.4)	0.7 (4.2)	15.1 (4.0)	15.2 (4.0)	0.1 (3.8)	11.9 (4.7)	12.6 (4.1)	0.7 (3.4)

*Higher scores indicate worse health for MLwHF, and better well-being for Spiritual Quality of Life.
[†]Difference between baseline and follow-up scores, negative values indicate improvement for MLwHF, whereas positive values indicate improvement for Spiritual Quality of Life.

sociation with QOL. The association between change scores and time interval between assessments was nonlinear, and thus, the time interval variable was dichotomized into more than 163 days versus 163 days or less. This cutoff was chosen because the protocol required a follow-up assessment by week 19 (133 days), and we allowed another 30 days for delays. The rationale was that a greater time interval might indicate noncompliance, illness, or other unknown factors correlated with change scores. Controlling for time interval between assessments also serves to account for the natural progression of CHF.

The regression analysis results are listed in Table A3-3. The RR group had significantly better adjusted mean change scores than did the UC group in the peace subscale of the spiritual QOL measure (2.73 points higher, SE = 1.17, p = 0.02), whereas no significant difference was observed between EDU and UC groups. The RR patients also had a better adjusted mean change score, with marginal statistical significance (3.13 points, SE = 1.69, p = 0.07), than did UC patients in the emotional subscale of the disease-specific QOL measure. No statistically significant differences among the 3 groups in the adjusted change scores of the physical or faith subscales of the QOL measures were observed. Adjusted mean change scores of the emotional and peace subscales of the QOL measures of a reference patient in each group who had the mean value in the continuous covariates and in the reference group of the dichotomous covariates are displayed in Figure A3-2.

Analysis II Critique

Table A3-3 gives us some of the most helpful numbers to evaluate the outcome of this study. In the small print below the table are the p values. Some are <0.10 and thus would not be considered statistically significant. Those that are identified as <0.05, <0.001, and <0.01 are all statistically significant—that is, the differences reported are not due to chance. In each of these tables, the authors have reported the standard error (SE) or standard deviation (SD) next to actual results, and thus, we can judge whether there was a relatively large amount of variation in the number. This is a good way to report these data. If the number in parentheses is very large compared with the reported result, then variability may have affected the outcome. Reading the text and using the tables, the reader can see that the intervention was apparently linked to some improvements and not to others. It takes some effort, however, to link the findings to what they mean. We will look to the discussion to summarize the differences for us, but we can link their conclusions back to these numbers. This is where a power analysis would be helpful. If we knew that the sample had sufficient power to detect differences, we would be more confident accepting the findings that appear to represent that the intervention had no effect.

Table A3-3 Regression Analysis Results of Quality-of-Life Change Scores

| | Quality-of-Life Measures, β* (SE) | | | |
| | Minnesota Living with Heart Failure† | | Spiritual Scale‡ | |
Independent Variables	PH	EH	Peace	Faith
Group				
RR (N = 31)	−2.55 (2.45)	−3.13§ (1.69)	2.73§ (1.17)	0.14 (0.97)
EDU (N = 24)	−1.80 (2.71)	−1.57 (1.85)	1.94 (1.31)	0.31 (1.09)
UC¶ (N = 28)	...	...	...	...
Baseline score	−0.41# (0.10)	−0.46# (0.10)	−0.36# (0.08)	−0.36# (0.09)
Days between assessments >163 days				
Yes	2.40 (2.27)	3.72‖ (1.56)	−0.53 (1.06)	−0.05 (0.89)
No¶	...	...	...	...
Age	0.33** (0.11)	0.13 (0.08)	−0.11‖ (0.05)	−0.002 (0.04)
At least college education				
Yes	−0.96 (2.30)	0.45 (1.59)	0.12 (1.08)	−0.02 (0.91)
No¶	...	...	...	...
On salt-restricted diet				
Yes	1.49 (2.75)	−2.55 (1.89)	−1.19 (1.31)	−1.24 (1.08)
No¶	...	...	...	...
Receiving medication††				
Ace inhibitors	−0.91 (4.16)	−8.09** (2.83)	2.43 (1.95)	2.24 (1.60)
Angiotensin II inhibitors	−0.67 (5.72)	−11.63** (3.95)	5.64‖ (2.70)	3.93§ (2.23)
β-Blockers	−5.31 (3.46)	1.56 (2.41)	−0.90 (1.63)	−1.34 (1.35)
Diuretics	0.11 (2.44)	1.96 (1.68)	0.50 (1.14)	−0.67 (0.96)
Intercept	−8.14 (10.95)	1.96 (7.77)	15.78 (5.00)	5.73 (4.10)
R	0.34	0.40	0.33	0.29

*Regression coefficient β and its standard error.

†Disease-specific quality-of-life measure: Minnesota Living with Heart Failure Questionnaire: negative change scores indicate improvement. It includes 2 subscales: PH: physical health subscale; and EH: emotional health subscale.

‡The Functional Assessment of Chronic Illness Therapy—Spiritual Well-Being: positive change scores indicate improvement. It includes 2 subscales: Peace: peace subscale; and Faith: faith subscale.

§p < .10

‖p < .05

¶The reference group.

#P < .001.

**P < .01

††Percentage of days between 2 assessments testing each of the medications.

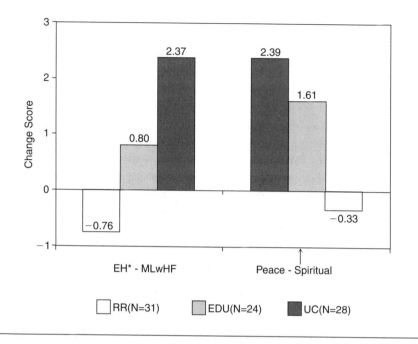

Figure A3-2   Emotional, peace-spiritual quality-of-life adjusted change score.
Adjusting for baseline scores, days between the assessments, age, education,
salt-restricted diet, and CHF medications; days between assessments of less
than 163 days, less than college education, no salt-restricted diet, and mean
value of all the other variables were used to calculate the adjusted change
score in each group.
*Comparison between RR and US groups: $P = .07$.
†Comparison between RR and UC groups: $P = .02$. EH-MLwHF indicates Emotional Health subscale in the Minnesota Living with Heart Failure Questionnaire:
negative values indicate improvement; peace-spiritual, peace subscale in the
spiritual scale: positive values indicate improvement; RR: relaxation response
group; EDU: cardiac education group; and UC: usual care group.

Intervention Compliance

Group attendance of RR and EDU patients was fairly good. Among the 31
RR patients who completed baseline and follow-up QOL measures, average attendance was 11 sessions with an SD of 4 and ranged from 2 to 16 sessions
with two thirds of patients attending at least 10 sessions. Similarly, the 24 EDU
patients who completed baseline and follow-up QOL measures attended 10
sessions on average (SD = 5) and ranged from 0 (2 patients) to 15 sessions
with two thirds attending at least 10. Home practice was also reasonably good.

The 31 RR patients practiced an average of 70 days (SD of 41 days) between the 2 QOL assessments (average interval = 169 days). Practice averaged 5.3 twenty-minute sessions per week (SD = 3.6) during this period. There was a small, but not statistically significant, positive correlation between the amount of practice and the peace QOL change scores (r = 0.22, p = 0.23) for the 31 RR patients.

Participants Characteristics

Only 75 (24 RR, 25 EDU, and 26 UC) of the 95 enrolled patients completed baseline bicycle tests. A protocol change early in the study allowed patients who could not perform the test (for reasons such as having difficulty keeping the mouthpiece in during the test, knee problems, and having a wheelchair) to be enrolled in the study. This protocol change increased recruitment.[15] Patients who took the baseline bicycle test were similar to those who did not in age, LVEF, and comorbidity as measured by Charlson's index. Patients who took the baseline test, however, had better scores in the QOL scales, but differences reached statistical significance of at least 5% only in the emotional subscale of MLwHF.

Among the 75 patients who completed the baseline bicycle test, 50 (16 RR, 16 EDU, and 18 UC) completed follow-up tests. Poor health, the unavailability of the exercise physiologist or a cardiologist, and malfunctioning equipment prevented some follow-up tests. No significant difference in the baseline bicycle test results was observed between the 50 patients who took both tests and the 25 patients who took only the baseline test. A complete data analysis approach on 50 patients with both baseline and follow-up bicycle test results was therefore used.[29]

Group Comparison

Following the same rationale as QOL measures, we controlled for baseline measures, time between assessments, age, education, diet, and CHF medications when making group comparison in the change values of the 3 parameters of the bicycle test. No significant difference was observed among the 3 groups in the adjusted change values of VO_2max, total exercise time, and workload. The adjusted change values of the 3 parameters from the bicycle test of a reference patient in each study group are displayed in Figure A3-3.

DISCUSSION

In this randomized trial of an RR intervention for patients with CHF, we enrolled 95 patients and completed follow-up QOL measures for 83 (87%). No significant dropout bias was observed. Analysis of the 83 patients revealed

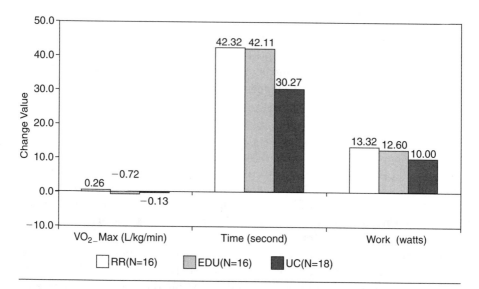

Figure A3-3 Exercise bicycle test results: Adjusted change value. Adjusting for baseline values, days between the assessments, age, education, salt-restricted diet, and CHF medications; days between assessments of less than 163 days, less than college education, no salt-restricted diet, and mean value of all the other variables were used to calculate the adjusted change value in each group. Positive values indicate improvement; no statistically significant difference among the 3 study groups. VO_2max indicates peak oxygen consumption; time: total exercise time; work: workload; RR: relaxation response group; EDU: cardiac education group; and UC: usual care group.

significant study intervention effects in the spiritual domains of the QOL measures as indicated in the adjusted change scores. There was also some trend of the intervention effect in the emotional QOL.

These findings of the intervention effect on spiritual and emotional QOL have important implication for the care of CHF patients. Advanced heart failure has been termed "heart cancer" because of its incurable condition associated with an inexorable decline in functional status. Despite advances in pharmacologic therapies, patient morbidity and mortality remain high and CHF patients experience serious decline in their QOL. A nonpharmaceutical intervention such as the RR that can improve QOL of these patients, particularly in the spiritual and emotional domains, is valuable. The important role of spirituality in health and medical care has been highlighted in the literature.[30,31] Improving emotional well-being can also contribute to the overall well-being particularly for CHF patients. Our study results suggest that integrating the RR training into CHF healthcare settings such as cardiac rehabilitation or heart failure programs may have beneficial effects.

This trial did not show statistically significant intervention effects on physical QOL or exercise capacity. Statistical nonsignificance might be due to (1) the size of the trial (limiting statistical power to detect small effect sizes), particularly for exercise test; (2) the use of standardized QOL scales (not capturing physical improvements experienced by study participants); and (3) the relatively short intervention and imperfect compliance. Studies demonstrating physiologic effects from meditation usually included long-time practitioners or longer interventions.[32–34]

Study limitations stem from the population: all veterans, nearly all men and with moderate CHF severity. The results are thus not generalizable to nonveterans, women, or patients with mild or severe CHF.

CONCLUSIONS CRITIQUE

The authors do a good job of summarizing the statistical findings so that we can easily find the most important conclusions from this study. The information we need to determine the external validity of the study is also explicit. The authors are straightforward in describing the groups for whom these results are relevant.

This randomized trial is one of the very few to evaluate an RR in CHF patients. The strength of this trial is the inclusion of a comparison intervention group. Future larger trials with longer interventions can serve to confirm the intervention effects on emotional and spiritual health and to better assess the effect of the RR on physical health and exercise capacity.

ACKNOWLEDGMENTS

This research was supported by the Department of Veterans Affairs, Health Services Research and Development grant (IIR 99–241). The views expressed in this article are those of the authors and do not necessarily represent the views of the Department of Veterans Affairs. We are indebted to the veterans who volunteered to participate in the study. We also thank all the personnel who contributed their time to this project in recruitment, intervention, data management, and data analysis.

REFERENCES

1. Eisenberg DM, Davis RB, Ettner SL, et al. Trends in alternative medicine use in the United States, 1990–1997: results of a follow-up national survey. *JAMA* 1998;280:1569–1575.
2. Benson H, Beary J, Carol M. The relaxation response. *Psychiatry.* 1974;37:37–46.
3. Benson H. *The Relaxation Response.* New York: Avon Books; 1975.
4. Beary J, Benson H. A simple psychophysiologic technique which elicits the hypometabolic changes of the relaxation response. *Psychosom Med* 1974;36:115–120.
5. Eppley KR, Abrams AJ, Shear J. Differential effects of relaxation techniques on trait anxiety: a meta-analysis. *J Clin Psychol* 1989;45:957–974
6. Kabat-Zinn J, Massion AO, Kristeller J, et al. Effectiveness of a meditation-based stress reduction program in the treatment of anxiety disorders. *Am J Psychiatry* 1992;149:936–943.
7. Miller JJ, Fletcher K, Kabat-Zinn J. Three-year follow-up and clinical implications of a mindfulness meditation-based stress reduction intervention in the treatment of anxiety disorders. *Gen Hosp Psychiatry* 1995;17:192–200.
8. Taylor DN. Effects of a behavioral stress-management program on anxiety, mood, self-esteem, and T-cell count in HIV positive men. *Psychol Rep* 1995;76:451–457.
9. Zamarra JW, Schneider RH, Besseghini I, Robinson DK, Salerno JW. Usefulness of the transcendental meditation program in the treatment of patients with coronary artery disease. *Am J Cardiol* 1996;77:867–870.
10. Alexander CN, Schneider RH, Staggers F, et al. Trial of stress reduction for hypertension in older African Americans. II. Sex and risk subgroup analysis. *Hypertension* 1996;28:228–237. 11. 11. Schneider RH, Staggers F, Alxander CN, et al. A randomized controlled trial of stress reduction for hypertension in older African Americans. *Hypertension* 1995;26:820–827.
12. Luskin F, Reitz M, Newell K, Quinn TG, Haskell W. A controlled pilot study of stress management training of elderly patients with congestive heart failure. *Prev Cardiol* 2002;5:168–172.
13. Klaus LMD, Beniaminovitz AMD, Choi LBA, et al. Pilot study of guided imagery use in patients with severe heart failure. *Am J Cardiol* 2000;86:101–104.
14. Chang B-H, Jones D, Hendricks A, Boehmer U, LoCastro J, Slawsky M. Relaxation response for VA patients with congestive heart failure: results from a qualitative study within a clinical trial. *Prev Cardiol* 2004;7:64–70.
15. Chang B-H, Hendricks A, Slawsky M, LoCastro J. Patient recruitment to a randomized clinical trial of behavioral therapy for chronic heart failure. *BMC Med Res Methodol* 2004;4:8.

16. Benson H. The Mind Body Medical Institute. Available at http://www.mbmi.org. Accessed April 15, 2005.

17. Mason J. *Guide to Stress Reduction*. Berkeley, Calif: Celestial Arts; 1997. Available at www.dstress.com. Accessed April 15, 2005.

18. Rector SR, Kubo SH, Cohn JN. Validity of the Minnesota Living with Heart Failure Questionnaire as a measure of therapeutic response to enalapril or placebo. *Am J Cardiol* 1993;71:1106–1107.

19. Brady MJ, Peterman AH, Fitchett G, Mo M, Cella D. A case for including spirituality in quality of life measurement in oncology. *Psycho-Oncology* 1999;8:417–428.

20. Jenkinson C, Jenkinson D, Shepperd S, Layte R, Petersen S. Evaluation of treatment for congestive heart failure in patients aged 60 years and older using generic measures of health status (SF-36 and COOP charts). *Age Aging* 1997;26:7–13.

21. Guyatt GH. Measurement of health-related quality of life in heart failure. *J Am Coll Cardiol* 1993;22:185A–191A.

22. Cohen-Solal A, Zannad F, Kayanakis JG, Guerets P, Aupetit JF, Kolsky H. Multicentre study of the determination of peak oxygen uptake and ventilatory threshold during bicycle exercise in chronic heart failure. *Eur Heart J* 1991;12:1055–1063.

23. Metra M, Nodari S, Raccagni D, et al. Maximal and submaximal exercise testing in heart failure. *J Pharmacol* 1998;32:S36–S45.

24. Deyo RA, Cherkin DC, Ciol MA. Adapting a clinical comorbidity index for use with ICD-9-CM administrative databases. *J Clin Epidemiol* 1992;45:613–619.

25. Charlson ME, Pompei P, Ales KL, MacKenzie CR. A new method of classifying prognostic comorbidity in longitudinal studies: development and validation. *J Chronic Dis* 1987;40:373–383.

26. Sherbourne CD, Stewart AL. The MOS Social Support Survey. *Soc Sci Med* 1991;32:705–714.

27. Washburn RA, McAuley E, Katula SL, Mihalko SL, Boileau RA. The Physical Activity Scale for the Elderly (PASE): evidence for validity. *J Clin Epidemiol* 1999;52:643–651.

28. Geoffrey K. Comparisons among treatment means. In: *Design and Analysis: A Researcher's Handbook*. Englewood Cliffs, NJ: Prentice-Hall; 1973:85–103.

29. Rubin DB. Inference and missing data. *Biometrika* 1976;63:581–592.

30. Chally PS, Carlson JM. Spirituality, rehabilitation, and aging: a literature review. *Arch Phys Med Rehabil* 2004;85:560–565.

31. Koenig HG, Idler E, Kasl S, et al. Religion, spirituality, and medicine: a rebuttal to skeptics [editorial]. *Int J Psychiatry Med* 1999;29:123–131.

32. Cunningham C, Brown S, Kaski JC. Effects of transcendental meditation on symptoms and electrocardiographic changes in patients with cardiac syndrome. *Am J Cardiol* 2000;85:653–655, A10.
33. Brooks JS, Scarano T. Transcendental meditation in the treatment of post-Vietnam adjustment. *J Counsel Dev* 1985;64:212–215.
34. Lazar S, Bush G, Gollub RL, Fricchione GL, Khalsa G, Benson H. Functional brain mapping of the relaxation response and meditation. *Neuro Report* 2000;11:1581–1585.

Checklist for Evaluating a Research Study

_____ The purpose of the study is explicitly stated.

_____ The introduction provides support for the importance of the study.

_____ The research problem has significance for your clinical practice.

_____ The research question is appropriate, refined, and focuses on a single concept.

_____ Hypotheses are written appropriately for each inferential statistical test.

_____ The research question includes sufficient detail to identify _who_ is the population, _what_ will be measured, _how_ it will be measured, and _when_ it will be measured.

_____ The literature review relies primarily on the most recent studies.

_____ All or most of the major studies related to the topic of interest are included.

_____ The literature review can be linked directly and indirectly to the research question.

_____ The review provides support for the importance of the study.

_____ The review is unbiased and includes both conclusive _and_ inconsistent findings.

_____ The author's opinion is virtually undetectable in the literature review.

_____ The review is organized so that a logical unfolding of ideas is apparent.

_____ The review ends with a summary of the most important knowledge on the topic.

_____ The design is clearly identified.

_____ A rationale is provided for the choice of a design, and it is linked to the research question.

_____ A specific procedure is described for the application of the treatment or intervention.

_____ Instruments and measures are described objectively.

_____ The reliability of the instrumentation is described, and supporting statistics are provided.

_____ The validity of the instrumentation is described, and supporting statistics are provided.

_____ A detailed protocol for the use of each instrument is described.

_____ Threats to internal validity are identified and controlled.

_____ Researcher bias and treatment effects are controlled by blinding.

_____ The target population is clearly identified.

_____ Inclusion criteria are specific and objective.

_____ Exclusion criteria are specified as appropriate to control extraneous variables.

_____ Procedures for selecting the sample are specified (if not, assume a convenience sample).

_____ Sampling procedures are likely to produce a representative sample.

_____ Potential for sampling bias has been identified and controlled by the researcher.

_____ The sample is unaffected by common sources of bias such as homogeneity, nonresponse, and systematic attrition.

_____ The sample is of adequate size.

_____ Power analysis is conducted and reported and is at least 80% (unnecessary if all results were statistically significant).

_____ Descriptive statistics were reported for the sample.

_____ Tests for group equivalency were conducted and revealed no significant differences.

_____ P values were reported and were less than 0.05 for those described as significant.

_____ The right tests were used for the research question and level of measurement.

_____ Confidence intervals were reported that represented an acceptable level of precision.

_____ Effect size was calculated and reported and was clinically meaningful.

_____ This sample could reasonably be expected to represent my patients and settings.

_____ The setting for the study is similar to mine in key characteristics such as level of care, type of unit, and geographic locale.

A Bedside Science Research Flow Sheet

RESEARCH PROCESS

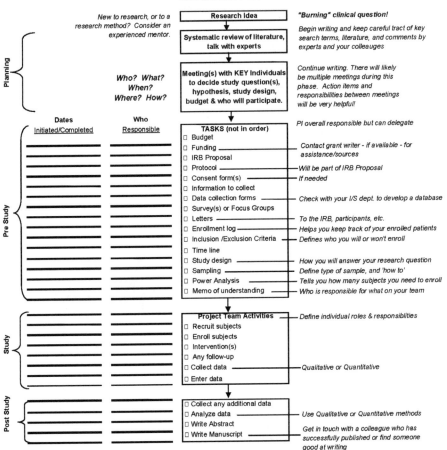

New to research, or to a research method? Consider an experienced mentor.

Research Idea — *"Burning" clinical question!*

Systematic review of literature, talk with experts — *Begin writing and keep careful tract of key search terms, literature, and comments by experts and your colleauges*

Who? What? When? Where? How?

Meeting(s) with KEY Individuals to decide study question(s), hypothesis, study design, budget & who will participate. — *Continue writing. There will likely be multiple meetings during this phase. Action items and responsibilities between meetings will be very helpful!*

Dates Initiated/Completed	Who Responsible

PI overall responsible but can delegate

Planning

Pre Study

TASKS (not in order)
- ☐ Budget
- ☐ Funding — *Contact grant writer - if available - for assistance/sources*
- ☐ IRB Proposal
- ☐ Protocol — *Will be part of IRB Proposal*
- ☐ Consent form(s) — *If needed*
- ☐ Information to collect
- ☐ Data collection forms — *Check with your I/S dept. to develop a database*
- ☐ Survey(s) or Focus Groups
- ☐ Letters — *To the IRB, participants, etc.*
- ☐ Enrollment log — *Helps you keep track of your enrolled patients*
- ☐ Inclusion /Exclusion Criteria — *Defines who you will or won't enroll*
- ☐ Time line
- ☐ Study design — *How you will answer your research question*
- ☐ Sampling — *Define type of sample, and 'how to'*
- ☐ Power Analysis — *Tells you how many subjects you need to enroll*
- ☐ Memo of understanding — *Who is responsible for what on your team*

Study

Project Team Activities — *Define individual roles & responsiblities*
- ☐ Recruit subjects
- ☐ Enroll subjects
- ☐ Intervention(s)
- ☐ Any follow-up
- ☐ Collect data — *Qualitative or Quantitative*
- ☐ Enter data

Post Study

- ☐ Collect any additional data
- ☐ Analyze data — *Use Qualitative or Quantitative methods*
- ☐ Write Abstract
- ☐ Write Manuscript — *Get in touch with a colleague who has successfully published or find someone good at writing*

Definitions:

PI: Principal Investigator. Team leader and person who makes sure all study pieces are organized & completed. Legally responsible for project.

Co-PI: Shares PI responsibilities. Commits to specific tasks and/or activities.

Co-Investigators: Actively involved in this project. Commits to specific tasks and/or activities.

Study Coordinators: Orchestrates all important project activities (usually involved with large, complex studies).

Scientist: Experienced researcher who can serve as a mentor if needed, will be a co-investigator, and will be actively involved throughout project. She/he will provide expert research direction /advice and work directly with PI and study team.

Statistician/Biostatistician: Can provide guidance on your hypothesis, study design, type of statistical tests to use, power and sample size, and all other statistical issues.

Study Team: May consist of important individuals NOT on investigative team -- yet key to getting this project done. Commits to specific tasks and/or activities.

Index

serving on, 9
soliciting organizational commitment,
     17–18, 75–90
     ethical issues and IRB procedures, 77–81
resources, soliciting, 17–18, 85–87
     where to find resources, 88–89
resources for systematic reviews, 58–61
response rates, 144, 193, 198
results section, research abstracts, 217
retrospective studies, 41
     power calculation, 142
review process for publication, 228
reviewing research literature, 8–9, 16, 51–74
     for bedside scientist projects, 65–68
     case study (MTBI treatment protocol),
          70–73
     checklist for, 74, 263–264
     defining research questions, 35, 40
     example of, 243–262
     external validity, checking, 104, 186
     finding surveys, 195
     guideline development, 54–56
     internal validity, judging, 65
     looking for existing evidence-based guide-
          lines, 53
     methodology, finding, 100
     numbers in, evaluating, 164
     resources for, 88
     statistical results, looking for, 145
     surveys and qualitative research, evaluating,
          212
     systematic reviews, 16, 57–65
          focusing literature, 62–64
          judging methodologic quality, 64–65, 121
          research methods and, 94
          research questions vs., 15, 57–58
          resources for, 58–62

S

sample size, 22, 131–133, 142–144
     ordinal data and, 153
     qualitative studies, 201
sampling bias, 125. *See also* selection bias
sampling error, 125, 146
sampling strategies, 20–22, 123–138
     checklist for, 138
     controlling bias, 98, 125–127
     examples of, 133–138
          topical anesthetics (case study), 116
     external validity and, 170
     how to evaluate (example), 247

numeric descriptions of samples, 141–146
obtaining information about samples, 127
power calculation, 127, 129, 131–133, 142
     survey research, 193
qualitative studies, 200–201, 204
quality of, 65
selection bias, 95, 124–125
     controlling, 125–127
     from convenience sampling, 130
     external validity and, 169
     qualitative studies, 203
size of sample, 22, 131–133, 142–144
     ordinal data and, 153
     qualitative studies, 201
subject variability, 108–110
survey research, 193
saturation (sufficient sample size), 201
scale questions (surveys), 197
scaled (interval) data, 152, 154
scanning research literature, 8–9, 16, 51–74.
          See also systematic reviews
     for bedside scientist projects, 65–68
     case study (MTBI treatment protocol),
          70–73
     checklist for, 74, 263–264
     defining research questions, 35, 40
     example of, 243–262
     external validity, checking, 104, 186
     finding surveys, 195
     guideline development, 54–56
     internal validity, judging, 65
     looking for existing evidence-based guide-
          lines, 53
     methodology, finding, 100
     numbers in, evaluating, 164
     resources for, 88
     statistical results, looking for, 145
     surveys and qualitative research, evaluating,
          212
scientific evidence
     existing, looking for, 53. *See also* literature
          reviews
     guideline development, 54–56
     rating schemes, 54–55
     role of, 3–6
     survey and qualitative designs, 191–192
scope statement, 54
screening search results, 62–64
search strategy, 54, 58–61
     databases, 62
     screening process, 62–64